METHODS IN MOLECULAR BIOLOGY

Series Editor
John M. Walker
School of Life and Medical Sciences
University of Hertfordshire
Hatfield, Hertfordshire, AL10 9AB, UK

For further volumes:
http://www.springer.com/series/7651

ELISA

Methods and Protocols

Edited by

Robert Hnasko

Agricultural Research Service (ARS), U.S. Department of Agriculture, Albany, CA, USA

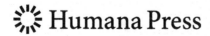

Editor
Robert Hnasko
Agricultural Research Service (ARS)
U.S. Department of Agriculture
Albany, CA, USA

ISSN 1064-3745   ISSN 1940-6029   (electronic)
Methods in Molecular Biology
ISBN 978-1-4939-2741-8   ISBN 978-1-4939-2742-5   (eBook)
DOI 10.1007/978-1-4939-2742-5

Library of Congress Control Number: 2015943593

Springer New York Heidelberg Dordrecht London

Cover illustration: Rendered three dimensional image of immunoglobulin (IgG1) protein as space filled and ribbon structure. Coordinates for IgG1 obtained from pdb1igy.pdb (Harris LJ, et al. J. Mol. Biol. 1998;275:861–872). Image by Robert Hnasko.

Printed on acid-free paper

Humana Press is a brand of Springer
Springer Science+Business Media LLC New York is part of Springer Science+Business Media (www.springer.com)

Preface

This book is intended as a practical biochemical guide to the Enzyme-Linked Immunosorbent Assay (ELISA) used to detect a target substance in a liquid sample. The ELISA is an important and widely used diagnostic tool in medicine, animal health, botany, and quality assurance processes in food and beverage production. The adoption of the ELISA by these industries is in part driven by the sensitivity and selectivity by which the assay can detect a desired target analyte along with it potential for standardization, automation, and economy of cost. The component parts of the ELISA are well suited for commercialization and adaptable for target detection using a diverse range of platforms.

The antibody is central to the performance of an ELISA providing the basis of analyte selection and detection. It is the interaction of antibody with analyte under defined conditions that dictates the outcome of the ELISA, and deviations in those conditions will impact assay performance. The aim of this manual is to provide the reader an overview of ELISA techniques and their potential application along with the technical aptitude necessary to design, run, and evaluate these immunoassays for the detection and quantitation of target analytes in solution.

The origin of a given protocol is difficult to determine and appropriate references are given when possible. Yet there will be many omissions as the pages of these protocols, derived from use in our laboratories, pass through the many hands of revision and refinement. No protocol is definitive and success often depends on the qualities of the antibodies and samples.

This book begins with an introductory chapter that is intended to orient the reader on the basic structure and function of immunoglobulins and their fragments. Arguably the antibody is the most important component of any immunoassay, and the second chapter in this book outlines the methodology to generate monoclonal antibodies using hybridoma technology. It is intended to provide the reader with an appreciation of how one can use hybridoma technology to generate and select for monoclonal antibodies that best meet the criteria of a given immunoassay. It should impress upon the immunoassay developer the value of an unlimited source of a stable characterized antibody and its commercial potential. The third chapter provides the general methods used to purify antibodies, and the fourth chapter provides one example of how to successfully conjugate an antibody to the enzymatic reporter horseradish peroxidase (HRP). In subsequent chapters these authors demonstrate how to creatively use the properties of the antibody to identify, localize, and quantify target analytes to answer questions and resolve problems. The reader will learn how to use a variety of immunoassay strategies, reporters, and detection systems that will undoubtedly facilitate their efforts to gain answers to their own questions. It is the goal of this book to provide the technical information necessary for the reader to successfully use the immunoassay as part of the discovery process.

Albany, CA, USA *Robert Hnasko*

Contents

Contributors

SONCHITA BAGCHI • *Department of Neuroscience, Uppsala biomedicinska centrum BMC, Uppsala University, Uppsala, Sweden*

DANIELA BOASSA • *National Center for Microscopy and Imaging Research and Center for Research on Biological Systems, University of California, San Diego, La Jolla, CA, USA*

M. LUIS CARBONELL • *MagArray Inc., Milpitas, CA, USA*

J. MARK CARTER • *Agricultural Research Service, U.S. Department of Agriculture, Albany, CA, USA*

SREEDEVI CHENNURU • *College of Veterinary Science, Sri Venkateswara Veterinary University, Proddatur, India*

KATHRYN H. CHING • *Crystal Bioscience, Emeryville, CA, USA*

LAURIE M. CLOTILDE • *MagArray Inc, Milpitas, CA, USA*

LAUREN FAGET • *Department of Neurosciences, School of Medicine, University of California San Diego (UCSD), La Jolla, CA, USA*

ROBERT FREDRIKSSON • *Department of Neuroscience, Uppsala biomedicinska centrum BMC, Uppsala University, Uppsala, Sweden*

XIAOHUA HE • *Foodborne Toxin Detection and Prevention Research Unit (FTDP), Agricultural Research Service (ARS), Pacific West Area (PWA), Western Regional Research Center (WRRC), United States Department of Agriculture (USDA), Albany, CA, USA*

THOMAS S. HNASKO • *Department of Neurosciences, School of Medicine, University of California San Diego (UCSD), La Jolla, CA, USA*

ROBERT M. HNASKO • *Produce Safety and Microbiology Unit (PSM), Agricultural Research Service (ARS), Pacific West Area (PWA), Western Regional Research Center (WRRC), United States Department of Agriculture (USDA), Albany, CA, USA*

MIKKI LARNER • *Plasmatreat USA Inc., Belmont, CA, USA*

ANDREW LIN • *United States Food and Drug Administration (FDA), Alameda, CA, USA*

ALICE V. LIN • *Produce Safety and Microbiology Unit (PSM), Agricultural Research Service (ARS), Pacific West Area (PWA), Western Regional Research Center (WRRC), United States Department of Agriculture (USDA), Albany, CA, USA*

ROBERT S. MATSON • *QuantiScientifics LLC, Irvine, CA, USA*

JEFFERY A. MCGARVEY • *Foodborne Toxin Detection and Prevention Unit (FTDP), Agricultural Research Service (ARS), Pacific West Area (PWA), Western Regional Research Center (WRRC), United States Department of Agriculture (USDA), Albany, CA, USA*

MARCELO A. NAVARRETE • *Department of Hematology, Leiden University Medical Center, RC Leiden, The Netherlands; School of Medicine, University of Magallanes, Punta Arenas, Chile*

STEPHANIE A. PATFIELD • *Foodborne Toxin Detection and Prevention Research Unit (FTDP), Agricultural Research Service (ARS), Pacific West Area (PWA), Western Regional Research Center (WRRC), United States Department of Agriculture (USDA), Albany, CA, USA*

PANDURANGA RAO PAVULURI • *Ella foundation, Genome Valley, Turkapally, Hyderabad, Telangana, India*

KHOREN SAHAGIAN • *Plasmatreat USA Inc., Belmont, CA, USA*

ALEXANDRA SALVADOR • *Agricultural Research Service, U.S. Department of Agriculture, Albany, CA, USA*

LARRY H. STANKER • *Foodborne Toxin Detection and Prevention Unit (FTDP), Agricultural Research Service (ARS), Pacific West Area (PWA), Western Regional Research Center (WRRC), United States Department of Agriculture (USDA), Albany, CA, USA*

ÅSA WALLÉN-MACKENZIE • *Department of Neuroscience, Unit of Functional Neurobiology, Uppsala University, Uppsala, Sweden; Department of Comparative Physiology, Uppsala University, Uppsala, Sweden*

HENG YU • *MagArray Inc., Milpitas, CA, USA*

Chapter 1

The Biochemical Properties of Antibodies and Their Fragments

Robert M. Hnasko

Abstract

Immunoglobulins (Ig) or antibodies are powerful molecular recognition tools that can be used to identify minute quantities of a given target analyte. Their antigen-binding properties define both the sensitivity and selectivity of an immunoassay. Understanding the biochemical properties of this class of protein will provide users with the knowledge necessary to select the appropriate antibody composition to maximize immunoassay results. Here we define the general biochemical properties of antibodies and their similarities and differences, explain how these properties influence their functional relationship to an antigen target, and describe a method for the enzymatic fragmentation of antibodies into smaller functional parts.

Key words Immunoglobulins, Antibodies, Immunoassay, Polyclonal, Antiserum, Monoclonal, Immunogen, Antigen, Analyte, Epitope, Affinity

1 Introduction

The fundamental principle that governs the performance of an immunoassay is the binding of an antibody to a specific antigen to form an exclusive antibody-antigen complex. An antigen or immunogen is any substance that elicits the production of specific antibodies (immune response) in an animal. Any molecule can be considered an immunogen (protein, chemical, nucleic acid, sugar) if it generates an immune response. Molecules that are native to the animal ("self") are much less likely to induce an immune response than those that are naive or foreign ("non-self"). In general large molecules of high molecular weight function well as immunogens, whereas smaller molecules (drugs, peptides, lipids) require chemical coupling to larger carrier proteins such as keyhole limpet hemocyanin (KLH) or bovine serum albumin (BSA) to generate what is termed a hapten to elicit an immune response. The immune response itself is highly variable and depends on the properties of the antigen, the animal, and method of immunization. Experimentally immunogens are combined with an adjuvant

Robert Hnasko (ed.), *ELISA: Methods and Protocols*, Methods in Molecular Biology, vol. 1318,
DOI 10.1007/978-1-4939-2742-5_1, © Springer Science+Business Media New York 2015

to create an emulsion that is used for immunization to potentiate the immune response. Immunizations are usually repeated over the course of several weeks to maximize the production of specific antibodies circulating in the blood (titer).

The site on the antigen to which a complementary antibody specifically binds is termed an epitope. Antibody-epitope binding may be continuous or linear such as sequence string of amino acids or discontinuous or conformational where binding depends on the three-dimensional shape. Antibody-antigen binding requires that the epitope be available and in the right shape. A multitude of factors can influence epitope availability that include aggregation, masking, chemical fixation or reduction, and changes in pH that may impede or facilitate the non-covalent antibody-antigen binding. Antibody affinity describes the strength of interaction with the antigen at a single antigenic site. All antibody-antigen interactions are reversible governed by thermodynamic principles that are described by an affinity constant (K_A). Affinity constants for antibody-antigen binding vary widely and are influenced by temperature, pH, and solvent. Avidity is a measure of the overall stability of the antibody-antigen complex and is mediated by affinity, valence of both antigen and antibody, and the organization of the interacting parts. Together these factors determine the specificity and the probability that a particular antibody will interact with a specific antigen epitope. Cross-reactivity of an antibody refers to binding of an antibody to epitopes on other antigens caused by low avidity or occurrence of identical or similar epitopes on multiple antigens. Cross-reactivity occurs frequently in antigenic groups where chemical structures or amino acid sequences are evolutionarily conserved [1–3].

The antibody is the central component of an immunoassay that is used for the detection of a target antigen or analyte. Antibodies exhibit exquisite antigen-binding selectivity at the molecular level which has been exploited to generate probes for the sensitive detection of target analytes used in diagnostic applications. Understanding the characteristics of antibodies and the methods used in their production, purification, and modification is crucial to their use as molecular recognition tools.

Antibodies are glycoproteins produced by plasma cells that function to bind foreign or non-self molecules. In response to a foreign antigen, the host can produce a diverse array of antibodies that are structurally similar yet unique in their properties. Small differences in amino acid sequence result in diverse and distinct properties that mediate antigen-binding versatility, specificity, and biological activity.

The basic structure of all antibodies or immunoglobulins (Ig) is illustrated in Fig. 1. This includes a four-chain structure composed of two identical light chains (23 kDa) and two identical heavy chains (50–70 kDa) as their basic unit. Interchain disulfide

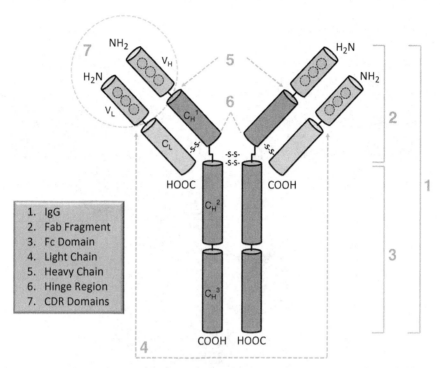

1. IgG
2. Fab Fragment
3. Fc Domain
4. Light Chain
5. Heavy Chain
6. Hinge Region
7. CDR Domains

Fig. 1 Structural domains of an immunoglobulin. A four-unit Y-structure is the basic organization of an immunoglobulin (150 kDa) molecule composed of two identical light chains (23 kDa) and two identical heavy chains (50–70 kDa) held together by interchain disulfide bonds (S–S). Each chain is divided by amino acid sequence into variable (V) and constant (C) regions. One variable and one constant region define the light chains (V_L and C_L). One variable (V_H) and three or four constant regions (C_H^{1-4}) define the heavy chains. A flexible hinge region is located between C_H^1 and C_H^2 on the heavy chains. The variable domains of both the light and heavy chains are further divided into three complementarity-determining regions (CDRs) separated by framework regions. The CDR or hypervariable regions of each light and heavy chain pair participate together to create the unique antigen-binding site. An intact native immunoglobulin or antibody is bivalent with each light and heavy chain CDR pair capable of binding to an antigen epitope. Specific cleavage of an antibody after C_H^1 at the hinge region can create two separate monovalent Fab fragments or a bivalent F(ab')2 if the interchain disulfide bond between the heavy chains remains intact. The remaining stalk of the molecule is referred to as the Fc effector domain (C_H^{2-4})

bonds hold together the heavy and light chains and the two heavy chains. Intra-chain disulfide bonds also contribute to the structure of each heavy and light chain [4]. Differences and similarities in the amino acid sequence of the heavy and light chain Ig divide these polypeptides into variable (V) and constant (C) regions. The light chain consists of one variable (V_L) and one constant domain (C_L), whereas the heavy chain consists of one variable (V_H) and three or four constant (C_H^1, C_H^2, C_H^3, C_H^4) domains. A hinge region between C_H^1 and C_H^2 is defined by molecular flexibility and is where the arms of the antibody form the Y. Although depicted as a linear Y-structure, the three-dimensional structural map reveals globular domains shaped by intra-chain disulfide bonds as

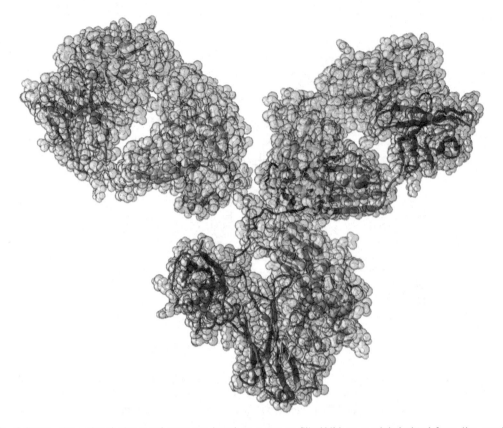

Fig. 2 Three-dimensional structural map rendered as a space-filled/ribbon model derived from the crystal structure of an immunoglobulin (IgG1; 1IGY.pbd)

illustrated in Fig. 2 as a space-filled/ribbon model derived from the crystal structure of an IgG1 [4]. Carbohydrates are attached to the C_H^2 domain in most antibodies but are not limited to this domain.

The variable domains show the most amino acid divergence within three regions called the hypervariable regions or complementarity-determining regions (CDRs) localized in both the heavy and light chains. It is the CDR domains of antibodies that are responsible for antigen-binding specificity. The regions between the CDRs in the V_L and V_H are called the framework region, and the similarities and differences within these regions, resulting from the product of distinct variable region genes, divide both the heavy and light chains into groups and subgroups [5, 6].

Immunoglobulins are divided into five classes (isotype) based on differences in amino acid sequences in the constant region of the heavy chain outlined in Table 1. IgG and IgA can be further divided into subclasses by additional differences in their constant region of the heavy chains. Yet all immunoglobulins within a class will have very similar sequences within this constant heavy chain region. Differences in the constant regions of the light chains

Table 1
Organization of immunoglobulin heavy chain class and light chain type

Class heavy chain (C_H^{1-3})	Subclass heavy chain (C_H^{1-3})
IgG	IgG1
	IgG2a
	IgG2b
	IgG3
IgA	IgA1
IgD	
IgE	
IgM	

Type light chain (C_L)	Subtype light chain (C_L)
Lambda	Lambda1
	Lambda2
	Lambda3
	Lambda4
Kappa	

define two light chain types (kappa and lambda), and further differences in the lambda chain result in identified lambda subtypes [7]. Table 2 illustrates the varied molecular weight, sedimentation coefficient, and pI of mouse antibody classes. The physiological properties of mouse antibody classes are outlined in Table 3.

Fragmentation of antibodies by limited proteolysis can be used to create different functional antibody units [8]. Digestion with papain disrupts the IgG before the interchain heavy chain disulfide bonds resulting in the generation of two identical Fab fragments each composed of the light chain and the V_H and C_H^1 domains of the heavy chain tethered together by the disulfide bridge (Fig. 3a). In addition an Fc domain is composed of the C_H^2 and C_H^3 domains of the two heavy chains held together by disulfide bonds. The Fc domain represents the effector functions of the Ig molecule that normally is involved in modulating immune cell function such as the fixation of complement which results in cell lysis or cell receptor binding. The activation of the antibody effector function normally requires prior antigen binding. The enzyme pepsin cleaves the Ig after the intra-chain disulfide bonds between the two heavy chains generating a F(ab')2 fragment composed of identical Fab-like fragments held together by a disulfide bond shown in Fig. 3b.

Table 2
Physicochemical properties of murine immunoglobulins

	MW (kDa)	Heavy chain	Heavy chain MW (kDa)	Light chain	Structure	Sedimentation coefficient	pI
IgA	170	α	70	λ or κ	Monomer—dimer	7S	4.0–7.0
IgD	180	δ	68	λ or κ	Monomer	7S	–
IgE	190	ε	80	λ or κ	Monomer	8S	–
IgG1	150	γ1	50	λ or κ	Monomer	7S	7.0–8.5
IgG2a	150	γ2a	50	λ or κ	Monomer	7S	6.5–7.5
IgG2b	150	γ2b	50	λ or κ	Monomer	7S	5.5–7.0
IgG3	150	γ3	50	λ or κ	Monomer	7S	–
IgM	900	μ	80	λ or κ	Pentamer	19S	4.5–7.0

Table 3
Biological concentration, distribution, and function of the immunoglobulin classes

Class	Serum (mg/mL)	% total Ig	% glycosylation	Distribution	Function
IgA	1–4	15	7–11	Intravascular and secretions	Protect mucus membranes
IgD	0–0.4	0.2	12–14	Lymphocyte surface	Unknown
IgE	10–400 ng/mL	0.002	12	Basophils and mast cells in secretions	Protect against parasites
IgG	5–12	75	2–3	Intra- and extravascular	Secondary response
IgM	0.5–2	10	12	Intravascular	Primary response

The Fc region of the protein is digested into small peptides and a pFc' domain. The disulfide bonds make the Ig sensitive to chemical reducing agents such as dithiothreitol (DTT) and 2-mercaptoethanol (2-ME) and effectively disrupt the inter- and intra-chain disulfide bonds and consequently antigen binding depicted in Fig. 3c.

Antigen binding is primarily mediated by the CDR regions of the variable domains of both the heavy and light chains (V_H and V_L) used to create the antibody combining site. Valency refers to this antigen-binding determinant composed of CDRs from both the V_H and V_L, and thus a single Ig is divalent, composed of two identical antigen-binding determinants. The generation of Fab fragments creates two monovalent antibody fragments, whereas the F(ab')2 retains a divalent binding characteristic [9, 10].

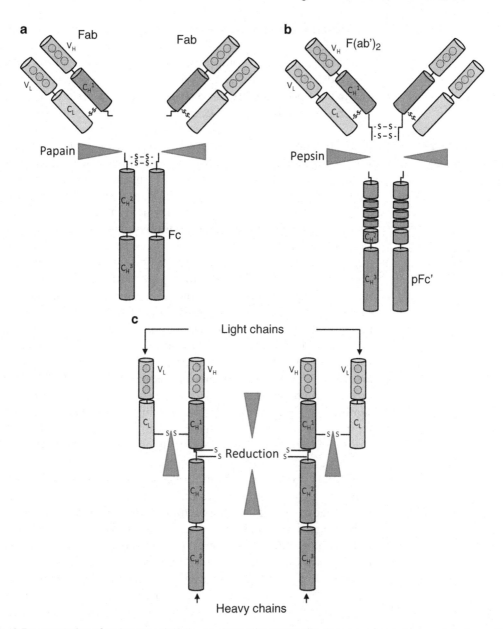

Fig. 3 Fragmentation of an immunoglobulin. (**a**) shows the enzymatic cleavage of an Ig by papain between C_H^1 and C_H^2 resulting in two monovalent Fab fragments and an Fc domain. (**b**) illustrates pepsin cleavage of an Ig after the disulfide bonds holding the two heavy chains together resulting in a divalent F(ab')2 fragment and pFc' domain. (**c**) shows chemical reduction of Ig with reducing agents such as DTT or 2-ME resulting in separation of the heavy and light chains by disruption of inter- and intra-chain disulfide bonds

Immunoglobulin names are based on class/subclass and type. Unless specifically stated, it should be assumed that an "antibody" is a heterogenous composition that includes a combination of class/subclass and type of immunoglobulin. Consider that each immunoglobulin in the mixture will have different antigen-binding properties and the user will have no knowledge of the ratio or composition of the antibodies present. Antisera or polyclonal antibodies will have this composition reflecting a pool of antibodies directed against an antigen. Monoclonal antibodies have a single defined antibody directed at a single antigen-determining region, and the isotype is usually specified.

1.1 Polyclonal and Monoclonal Antibodies

It is important to differentiate between polyclonal and monoclonal antibodies experimentally in order to maximize their strengths and weaknesses for their application in immunoassays. Some of the major differences between monoclonal and polyclonal antibodies are outlined in Table 4. Many high-quality polyclonal antibodies have been generated for use in immunoassays by repeated immunization of animals with a specific immunogen. Serum is harvested during the peak of antibody production that can yield concentrations of 1–10 mg. The resulting polyclonal antiserum contains many different antibodies capable of binding an immunogen with varied affinity and avidity at a multitude of antigenic epitopes (poly meaning many). Use of polyclonal antiserum in an immunoassay can result in multiple antibodies binding at distinct epitopes on a single antigen which can be used to enhance target detection or isolation. This multiplicity provides added tolerance for an immunoassay where small changes in the antigen presentation may not significantly impact overall binding but consequently serves to limit the discrimination potential of an assay. Understanding the nature of the immunogen used to generate the polyclonal serum can be extremely useful in predicting cross-reactivity. Native or recombinant proteins as immunogens have a higher probability of generating polyclonal antiserum with cross-reactivity to other homologous protein family members. Peptide sequences used as immunogens that have been screened by database search to be unique have lower probability of generating cross-reactive antibodies but can generate antibodies to non-native structure or unavailable epitopes in the parent protein resulting in artifact or an inability to bind native protein. Many of these confounding attributes

Table 4
Differences between polyclonal (pAb) and monoclonal (mAb) antibodies

Polyclonal (pAb)	Monoclonal (mAb)
Recognize multiple epitopes on a single antigen	Recognize a single antigen epitope
Easy to generate in a variety of animal species	Specialize techniques to generate with most derived from mouse Ig
Finite quantity	Unlimited quantity
Can be cross-reactive	Highly specific

can be minimized by screening and selection processes of antibodies during or after production (*see* **Note 1**). For example, species cross-reactivity of polyclonal antiserum can be minimized by pre-absorption of antiserum with a cross-reactive species to deplete the pool of antibodies that would bind undesirably to that particular species.

Monoclonal antibodies (mono meaning one) represent a homogenous pool of identical antibodies which bind to a single antigenic epitope with a defined affinity and avidity. The homogeneity of the monoclonal antibody results in a high degree of specificity but often with a limited tolerance for changes in epitope. This allows for detection of subtle molecular changes between and within antigens but also makes the use of monoclonals more vulnerable to changes in assay conditions.

Normal serum contains ~10^{16} antibodies per milliliter, and these antibodies can be collected from experimental animals to identify, label, or separate molecules and cells. However the variability of antisera combined with its finite quantity can be disadvantageous when building an immunoassay. The advantage of a polyclonal antibody pool is there are numerous antibodies that can be used to bind a given target at different molecular sites. The disadvantage is that some or many of the antibodies in the pool may exhibit poor binding characteristics, whereas the desired antibody/s in the pool may only be present in limited quantity. Moreover polyclonal antibodies represent a limited commodity that will run out, and effort to generate new antisera will invariably result in a different pool of antibodies even with the same immunogen. Furthermore bioconjugation of polyclonal antibodies is confounded by the varied ratio and quantity of each within a given pool resulting in potentially varied results.

Monoclonal antibodies have the advantage of being a continuous renewable resource. Thus the characterized properties of a monoclonal antibody will not change over time, an important consideration in developing an immunoassay and technology transfer. Clear properties of a monoclonal antibody can be defined such as binding affinity (KD), isotype, epitope, and CDR domains. As monoclonal antibodies represent a homogenous pool, they are readily conjugated and can be easily characterized.

1.2 Enzymatic Fragmentation of Antibodies

Conventional methods for IgG fragmentation to a monovalent Fab fragment are carried out using papain digestion and bivalent F(ab')2 fragment using pepsin digestion. Papain proteolysis produces Fab fragments from all IgG subclasses and species, whereas pepsin is less universal. Alternate F(ab')2 fragmentation can be accomplished with those IgGs using the enzyme ficin and is particularly useful for mouse IgG1.

To achieve IgG fragmentation into monovalent Fab fragments, preliminary test should be used to determine optimal papain conditions (concentration and time) for IgG fragmentation prior to large-scale antibody digestion. Results of digestion should be compared by Coomassie staining following SDS-polyacrylamide gel electrophoresis to determine optimal conditions. Nonreduced IgG migrates to ~150 kDa, Fab fragments ~50 kDa, and Fc fragments ~27 kDa. Under reducing conditions (10 % 2-ME or DTT), IgG will migrate as two bands of ~50 and 25 kDa, Fab fragments will yield a doublet of ~23–25 kDa, and Fc fragments will migrate as a band ~26 kDa. The biochemical effect of papain cleavage and chemical reduction of IgG1 molecular weight following SDS-PAGE is illustrated in Fig. 4.

2   Materials

37 °C incubator or water bath.

Magnetic stir bar and mixer.

Timer.

1.5 mL microfuge tubes.

Centrifuge.

Rocking platform.

P200 pipette and tips.

Transfer pipette.

Purified IgG at 2 mg/mL in PBS.

Phosphate-buffered saline (PBS); pH 7.2.

0.5 M EDTA (disodium salt) stock in PBS.

Freshly prepared 1 M L-cysteine in PBS.

Papain enzyme (lyophilized powder) in freshly prepared PBS digestion buffer stored on ice (<4 h) containing 0.02 M EDTA (disodium salt) and 0.01 1 M L-cysteine.

Freshly prepare 0.3 M iodoacetamide from solid in PBS.

Immobilized protein-A agarose (6 % cross-linked). Gently mix protein-A agarose bead stock by swirling suspension (do not vortex) and transfer defined volume to a fresh tube using a wide-bore pipette. To remove preservatives, wash beads by dilution in PBS 1:5 swirl and then slow centrifugation for 5 min at $900 \times g$ in fixed angle rotor; repeat. Resuspend beads in PBS equivalent to initial volume taken from stock slurry ~50 %:

2-Mercaptoethanol (2-ME).

Reagents and equipment for gel electrophoresis of proteins.

Colloidal Coomassie brilliant blue (G-250). Suspend 0.5 g Coomassie G-250 dye in a glass bottle by dissolving in 494.2 mL

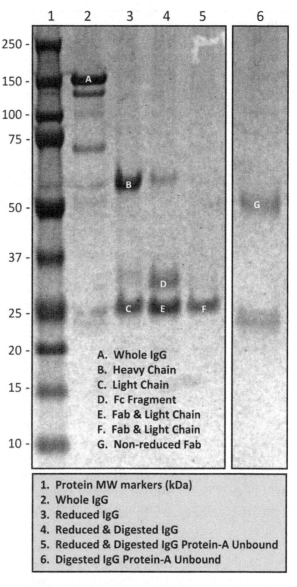

Fig. 4 Coomassie stained gel showing antibody fragmentation with papain after electrophoresis. *Lane 1* represents molecular weight protein ladder in kDa. *Lane 2* shows a banding pattern of native whole IgG with (**a**) denoting the intact 150 kDa antibody. *Lane 3* shows antibody separation into heavy (**b**) and light (**c**) chains following chemical reduction with 2-ME. *Lane 4* shows papain-digested Fc (**d**) and Fab (**e**) fragments in the presence of reducing agent. *Lane 5* shows protein-A purified Fab fragments with (**f**) and *Lane 6* without (**g**) chemical reduction

ultrapure water with 50 g ammonium sulfate and 5.8 mL phosphoric acid using a stir bar to create a stock solution. Freshly prepare working Coomassie G-250 solution by transferring 24 mL of well-mixed stock suspension to 6 mL of methanol. Mix and add enough to completely cover gel.

3 Methods

1. Prepare two papain solutions in 5 mL of digestion buffer at 100 and 20 μg/mL (*see* **Note 2**).

2. Number 12×1.5 mL microcentrifuge tubes and pipette 100 μL of 2 mg/mL purified IgG in PBS into each tube (*see* **Note 3**).

3. Mix the papain "suspensions" well by vortexing and then add 100 μL of 100 μg/mL papain to five tubes containing IgG and 100 μL of 20 μg/mL papain to the other five tubes containing IgG. In one of the two remaining control tubes, add 100 μL digestion buffer without papain and the other tube 100 μL of PBS (*see* **Note 4**).

4. Bring an incubator or water bath to 37 °C, set a timer, and begin incubating ten papain-containing tubes and the two control tubes. At 2, 5, 8, 18, and 24 h, remove one tube that contains papain at each concentration and add 40 μL of freshly prepared 300 mM iodoacetamide in PBS, vortex, and incubate for 30 min at room temperature to stop the enzymatic reaction (*see* **Note 5**).

5. Cleaved Fab fragments can be purified by binding residual intact antibodies and Fc fragments to immobilized protein-A. Using a transfer pipette, or a P200 pipette tip that has to be cut 1 cm from the bottom to create a wide-bore, transfer ~50 μl washed protein-A bead slurry per mg of digested antibody into a microfuge tube (*see* **Note 6**). Incubate with rocking for 20–30 min at room temperature, centrifuge the tubes at $900 \times g$ to pellet beads, transfer supernatants to a fresh tube, centrifuge at $3,000 \times g$, and harvest supernatants containing only Fab fragments (*see* **Note 7**).

6. Perform SDS-PAGE on digested antibody products and controls. Dilute 25 μl of digest (~20 μg) in sample buffer with and without 2-ME. Heat denature samples for 10 min and load on polyacrylamide gel and electrophorese.

7. Evaluate IgG digestion products by Coomassie protein stain (*see* **Note 8**). Remove gel after electrophoresis and incubate in ddH$_2$O with repeated rocking to remove SDS. Add working solution of Coomassie stain overnight at room temperature with rocking. Destain gel using repeated washes with ddH$_2$O to resolve protein bands. Evaluate stained gel for antibody fragmentation to identify optimal parameters for Fab fragmentation of target antibody (*see* **Note 9**).

4   Notes

1. The notion of "garbage in, garbage out" holds true for all those making antibodies. If the immunogen is impure or damaged by proteolytic fragmentation, the resulting antibodies generated merely reflect the immunogen. This is very evident when generating crude antiserum where antibodies generated against immunogen impurities are often the culprit behind nonspecific interactions. These antibodies can be minimized by postproduction purification methods. This is usually not possible when purchasing a small amount of expensive antiserum for evaluation. Consequently not all antisera are created equal and users may have to evaluate a number of vendors to find a source that works for their application. Monoclonal antibodies don't suffer this same fate as all the antibodies are identical and specific for a single epitope, whatever it may be. Commercial services that provide antibody generation often combine peptide immunogen production with antibody generation. Keep in mind that the titer guarantee is simply toward peptide detection and not the actual target of interest. You might get back antisera or monoclonal antibody that is fantastic at detecting the peptide but fails to detect the actual target analyte. Complex screening and selection strategies are often necessary to generate those high-value antibodies that perform well in immunoassays. Partner with laboratories that can improve the odds of generating a useful antibody reagent. If the intent is to building an immunoassay for a commercial application, it is highly recommended that the critical antibody component be renewable (monoclonal) and under your control (ownership or license).

2. Papain is a single-chain 23 kDa cysteine protease of the peptidase C1 family. Optimal activity is at pH 6–7. Papain is soluble in water at 10 mg/mL. The enzyme is prepared fresh by dissolving in 2× "digestion buffer" containing 10 mM L-cysteine and 20 mM EDTA for activation of enzymatic activity immediately prior to use in antibody fragmentation.

3. Inclusion of an established positive control antibody in which optimal parameters for digestion have been defined can be helpful to validate enzyme activity as an internal control to ensure proper performance and interpretation of results.

4. Ratio of enzyme/antibody is 1:100 and 1:20 with two control tubes used to evaluate the effect of digestion buffer alone on IgG and native IgG structure.

5. Iodoacetamide at the final concentration of 60 mM irreversibly inactivates papain.

6. To avoid bead shearing, use wide-bore tips and do not vortex; rather invert or swirl to mix. Wash the beads to remove preservative and any free unbound protein-A.

7. Residual intact antibody and the Fc fragments will bind the immobilized beads, and free Fab fragments will be unbound in the supernatants.

8. Coomassie blue is a reversible stain capable of detecting ~30 ng protein. This method is compatible with downstream mass spectrometry analysis.

9. Undigested nonreduced antibody will migrate to ~150 kDa, Fab ~50 kDa, and Fc ~27 kDa. Smaller bands may be present that represent other unimportant digestion products. Cysteine effects alone can result in a band at 120 kDa which would be observed in the no papain control samples. If this band is present, the digestion reaction should proceed until both the 150 and 120 kDa bands are both absent.

References

1. Elgert KD (1998) Antibody structure and function. In: Elgert KD (ed) Immunology: understanding the immune system. Wiley, New York, pp 58–78

2. Janeway CA Jr, Travers P, Walport M et al (2001) Immunobiology: the immune system in health and disease, 5th edn. Garland Science, New York

3. Male D, Brostoff J, Roth D, Roitt I (2012) Immunology, 8th edn. Elsevier, Philadelphia, PA

4. Harris LJ, Skaetsky E, McPherson A (1998) Crystallographic structure of an intact IgG1 monoclonal antibody. J Mol Biol 275:861–872

5. Davies DR, Chacko S (1993) Antibody structure. Acc Chem Res 26:421–427

6. Honjo T (1983) Immunoglobulin genes. Annu Rev Immunol 1:499–528

7. Blomberg B, Traunecker A, Eisen H, Tonegawa S (1981) Organization of four mouse lambda light chain immunoglobulin genes. Proc Natl Acad Sci U S A 78:3765–3769

8. Greenfield EA (2013) Antibodies: a laboratory manual, 2nd edn. Cold Spring Harbor Laboratory Press, Woodbury, NY

9. Schroeder HW Jr, Cavacini L (2010) Structure and function of immunoglobulins. J Allergy Clin Immunol 125:S41–S52

10. Wang W, Singh S, Zeng DL et al (2007) Antibody structure, instability, and formulation. J Pharm Sci 96:1–26

Chapter 2

Hybridoma Technology

Robert M. Hnasko and Larry H. Stanker

Abstract

The generation of hybridoma cell lines by the fusion of splenocytes from immunized mice with immortal myeloma cells is a well-established method for the production of monoclonal antibodies. Although other methods have emerged as an effective alternative for the generation of monoclonal antibodies, the use of hybridoma technology remains a viable technique that is accessible to a wide number of laboratories that perform basic cell biological research. Hybridoma technology represents a relatively simple procedure at minimal cost for the continuous production of native whole immunoglobulins. This chapter will describe the materials and methodologies needed for the successful generation of monoclonal antibody (mAb)-producing hybridoma cell lines against target antigens.

Key words Hybridoma, Myeloma, Monoclonal antibody, Antigen, Ascites, ELISA

1 Introduction

Hybridoma technology provides a useful means of generating monoclonal antibodies against any antigenic molecule. The production or isolation of a high-quality immunogen is the first step in the process. This can be accomplished by any number of methods that include: (1) chemical synthesis, (2) purification, (3) peptide synthesis, or (4) recombinant protein expression. An immunogen can be pure or crude and immunogenicity of the target will invariably influence the antigenic response following immunization. Consequently immunogenicity is determined empirically and is often facilitated by integration of large carrier molecules like keyhole limpet hemocyanin (KLH) or bovine serum albumin (BSA), adjuvant, animal, route, and schedule of immunizations. Provided that the immunogen elicits the desired immune response, the strategy used to identify or "screen" hybridomas for the desired monoclonal antibody (mAb) is essential for successful identification and isolation. Toward this aim it is necessary to define what type of mAb is to be identified and the appropriate hybridoma screening method devised to achieve the result.

Robert Hnasko (ed.), *ELISA: Methods and Protocols*, Methods in Molecular Biology, vol. 1318,
DOI 10.1007/978-1-4939-2742-5_2, © Springer Science+Business Media New York 2015

First consider the myeloma or hybrid cell line to be used as fusion partner from Table 1. These cell lines are all derived from a single parent Balb/c mouse lineage, yet by subcloning or fusion, they have evolved with different properties that influence cell fusion efficiency and production of extraneous antibodies [1–4]. We prefer lines that do not produce any immunoglobulins such as the P3X63-Ag8.653 and choose to immunize young postweaning (4–6 weeks) Balb/c mice to maintain isogenic compatibility to minimize potential rejection of cloned hybridoma cell lines used for in vivo production of ascites.

The immunogen will often define how the hybridoma screen will be performed. With purified or synthetic immunogens, efforts should be made to engineer the best tools to facilitate hybridoma screening for the target. For example, if one is to use the same synthetic peptide as the immunogen and the screening antigen, it is beneficial to use different carrier conjugates for immunization and screening to avoid isolation of antibodies against the carrier. In this scenario you might generate (1) a synthetic 20-mer peptide conjugated to KLH to serve as immunogen and (2) the same 20-mer peptide conjugated to BSA to serve as antigen for screening mAbs (*see* **Note 1**). Here you immunize with peptide-KLH and screen mAbs for binding to peptide-BSA immobilized on microtiter plates by indirect ELISA. An alternate scenario is that you immunize with a 20-mer peptide-KLH conjugate and screen against an immobilized crude extract containing the parent protein by iELISA. Similar strategies can be engineered for small chemical molecules or recombinant proteins expressed via DNA expression vectors containing terminal protein tags such as GST or SUMO. The basic principle is that if the immunogen is not "native" the antigen used in the hybridoma screen should differ to avoid isolating mAbs against undesired structures.

One of the simplest designs for isolating antigen uses the indirect ELISA (iELISA) where the target antigen is immobilized on plastic microtiter plates, hybridoma supernatants added to allow any mAb present to bind target, and an anti-mouse antibody conjugated to a reporter used to identify mAb binding to antigen. The commercial availability of isotype-specific secondary antibodies should be considered to avoid isolation of sticky nonspecific or low-affinity IgM antibodies (*see* **Note 2**). This approach for the identification of hybridomas producing target mAb is effective, but often the resulting antibody isolated fails to "capture" antigen in solution, an important requirement for at least one of the two antibodies used in the construction of a sandwich ELISA (sELISA). These "detector" types of antibodies are common and are often excellent at binding target antigen in a variety of immunoassay formats such as Western blot, immunohistochemistry, iELISA, or direct ELISA (dELISA). Equally they are usually suitable for use in sELISA as the detector mAb that is directly conjugated to a reporter.

Table 1
Myeloma cell lines and their properties used in the generation of hybridoma producing monoclonal antibodies

Cell Line	Chromosome#	Ig	Derivation	Origin	ATCC
P3X63-Ag8	65	IgG1, κ	MOPC-21	Kohler & Milstein	TIB-9
NS1-Ag4.1	65	κ (intracellular)	P3X27	Kohler & Milstein	TIB-18
P3X63-Ag8.653	58	NONE	P3X63-Ag8	Kearney	CRL-1580
SP2/0-Ag14	72	NONE	Hybridoma (P3X63-Ag8 x Balb/c)	Shulman & Kohler	CRL-1581
FO	72	NONE	Self fusion of SP2/0-Ag14 with Sendai virus	SF de St. Groth & Scheidegger	CRL-1646
S194/5.XXO.BU.1		IgA, κ (not secreted)	Balb/c	Hyman	TIB-20
MPC-11	62	IgG2b, κ	Balb/c	Laskov & Scharff	CCL-167
Y3.Ag1.2.3	39	κ	Lou rat S210 derivative	Galfre, Milstein & Wright	CRL-1631
NSO/u		NONE	NS1-Ag4.1	Clark & Milstein	Sigma-Aldrich #85110503

18

Most high-affinity in-solution capture antibodies are conformational, binding to discontinuous epitopes on the molecule. We believe that the immobilization of a protein antigen can deform the protein and skew the selection of mAbs toward those that best bind linear or continuous epitopes. To isolate a capture mAb usually requires a different hybridoma screening strategy. This usually requires the preexistence of a suitable "detector" antibody to create the pair (*see* **Note 3**). Often with novel antigens, these mAbs are not available and one might need to generate a detector mAb first before seeking a capture mAb. Other strategies can be devised that take advantage of recombinant DNA engineering or synthetic peptide chemistry. Here the integration of a protein tag (GST or SUMO) or biotin can be used with a corresponding tag-specific antibody to facilitate identification of a capture mAb.

One example of a basic screen for capture capable mAb for a protein might involve: (1) immobilizing an isotype-specific anti-mouse mAb on microtiter plates, (2) capturing mAb from hybridoma supernatants, (3) adding protein-tagged antigen in solution, and (4) adding non-murine polyclonal secondary detector antibody-conjugated reporter. Several alternatives can be devised that might include the use of an avidin reporter in place of a secondary antibody or immobilized avidin microtiter plates to capture and orient a biotinylated antigen followed by binding of hybridoma supernatant mAb and detection with an anti-mouse conjugated reporter.

It is important to have a hybridoma screening strategy defined to maximize the successful isolation of a mAb that binds target antigen and best meets the end-user need. Often a multitude of hybridomas will be cloned producing individual mAbs with unique antigen-binding properties that perform in some immunoassays and not others. Part of the characterization of an isolated mAb involves evaluation of cross-reactivity, species specificity, affinity, and immunoassay performance.

The basic workflow of generating a mAb using hybridoma technology is shown in Fig. 1 and includes: (1) immunogen design, production, and immunization, (2) cell fusion, (3) hybridoma selection with HAT, (4) hybridoma mAb screening, (5) cell cloning and expansion, and (6) ascite production [5–7]. After mice are immunized, those with the highest serum antibody titer to the antigen are euthanized and their spleen harvested (*see* **Note 4**). The final immunogen boost should be administered into the intraperitoneal cavity without adjuvant 3 days before the cell fusion (*see* **Note 5**).

Myeloma cells in culture should be split into fresh media 1 day before the fusion event to ensure log growth and maximal health (*see* **Note 6**). Myeloma cells are mixed with splenocytes in the presence of polyethylene glycol (PEG) to change membrane permeability and allow cell fusion. The cell fusion events are random

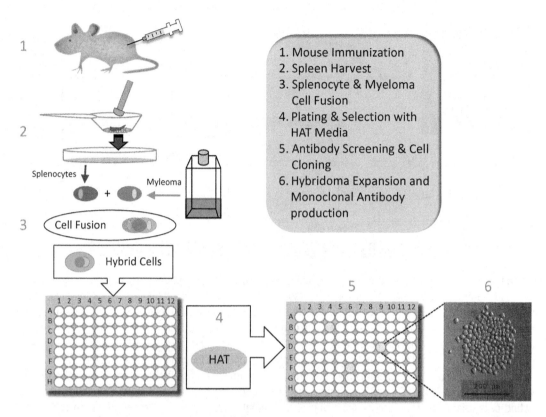

1. Mouse Immunization
2. Spleen Harvest
3. Splenocyte & Myeloma Cell Fusion
4. Plating & Selection with HAT Media
5. Antibody Screening & Cell Cloning
6. Hybridoma Expansion and Monoclonal Antibody production

Fig. 1 Schematic of hybridoma technology illustrating steps involved in the generation of a monoclonal antibody producing hybridoma cell line. *Step 1* is mouse immunization with defined antigen. *Step 2* spleen is harvested and splenocytes isolated. *Step 3* is splenocytes are fused with myeloma cells to generate hybrids. *Step 4* fused cells are cultured and hybrids selected by growth in HAT medium. *Step 5* surviving hybrid colonies are screened for production of antigen specific monoclonal antibody by immunoassay and cloned. *Step 6* hybridoma cell line established and expanded for production of antigen specific monoclonal antibody

and the culture will contain a mixture of single cells along with splenocyte-splenocyte, myeloma-myeloma, and hybrid myeloma-splenocyte.

Myeloma cells lack the enzyme hypoxanthine-guanine phosphoribosyltransferase (HGPRT) which prevents the cells from using the salvage pathway to synthesize purines as shown in Fig. 2. Myeloma cells grown in the presence of aminopterin, a folic acid analogue that blocks de novo cell biosynthesis of purines and pyrimidines necessary for DNA synthesis by inhibiting dihydrofolate reductase, will die even with the addition of salvage pathway precursors hypoxanthine and thymidine (HT) given their HGPRT status. Splenocytes express HGPRT and thymidine kinase (TK) enzymes and can utilize the salvage pathway for survival in the presence of aminopterin if supplied with hypoxanthine and thymidine (HT). Primary cells however are not immortal and will die off in time when grown in cell culture. Consequently hybrid cells that result from a fused myeloma-splenocyte retain the myeloma-contributed immortality and express HGPRT obtained from the

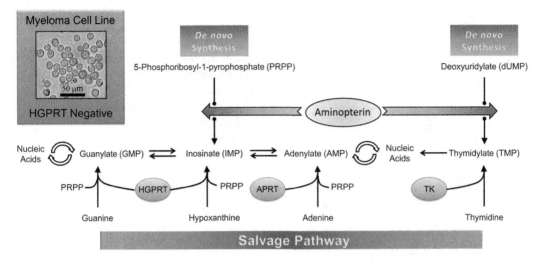

Fig. 2 Hybridoma survival and selection in cell culture is mediate by disruption of de novo nucleotide biosynthesis in the presence of salvage pathway precursors. Antifolates such as aminopterin block tetrahydrofolate reactivation which prevents de novo purine nucleotides (GMP, IMP, AMP) and thymidylate synthesis. In normal cells, the salvage pathways can be used in place of de novo synthesis to incorporate purine bases or nucleosides and thymidine into nucleic acids if the precursor hypoxanthine and thymidine (HT) are present. However, normal cells in culture will die out as they lack transformed properties for continued cell growth. Myeloma cells are transformed and are capable of continuous growth in culture, yet those that lack any of the salvage pathways enzymes (HGPRT, APRT or TK) will not survive in media containing antifolates. Splenocyte-myeloma hybrid cells retain the transformed phenotype of the parent myeloma for continued growth in culture and inherit the nucleotide salvage pathway from the splenocyte thereby survival and selection of hybridomas is achieved by growth in HAT supplemented medium. *HGPRT* hypoxanthine-guanine phosphoribosyltransferase, *APRT* adenine phosphoribosyltransferase, *TK* thymidine kinase, *HAT* hypoxanthine-aminopterin-thymidine

splenocyte allowing only the hybrid cells to survive and grow in HAT (hypoxanthine-aminopterin-thymidine)-supplemented medium.

The purpose of HAT medium is to (a) selectively kill unfused myeloma cells that would otherwise overgrow any fused hybrids generated and (b) eliminate any myeloma-myeloma hybrids that lack HGPRTase. HGPRT-positive splenocytes or splenocyte-splenocyte hybrids are not sensitive to HAT by means of salvage pathway support but as a primary cell have a finite lifespan and will die in culture over a short period of time. After HAT selection is complete (10–14 days), cell culture supernatants are screened for mAb, and those cells selected for expansion and cloning are passaged in medium containing hypoxanthine-thymidine (HT) without aminopterin before final expansion in normal hybridoma growth medium.

2 Materials

Laminar flow hood for sterile cell culture.

Autoclave.

Liquid aspirator.

Single and multichannel pipettes.

Clinical swinging bucket centrifuge.

37 °C water bath.

CO_2 incubator.

Hot plate.

Hemocytometer.

Timer.

Inverted phase contrast microscope.

Immunized mice that have been boosted with immunogen 3 days prior to the day of cell fusion.

Myeloma cell line, subcultured (split) the day before cell fusion to achieve $2–3 \times 10^5$ cells/mL.

Sterile stainless steel cell dissociation sieve with 100 mesh wire screen and pestle.

Sterile 5-mL disposable syringe.

Sterile cell scraper.

100-μm sterile cell strainer (BD Falcon).

500 mL Erlenmeyer flask.

200-mL glass beaker; filled with pre-warmed 37 °C water.

Red blood cell lysis buffer.

Hybridoma grade DMSO.

Sterile 100-mL solution basins.

Clear, sterile, 96-well, cell culture-treated, flat-bottom plates with lids.

Sterile surgical tools that include scissors and forceps.

70 % alcohol.

Sterile plastic petri dishes.

Sterile Pasteur pipettes.

5-, 10-, and 25-mL plastic disposable serological pipettes.

Sterile disposable polypropylene 15- and 50-mL conical tubes with screw top lid.

Solid polyethylene glycol (3,000–3,700 PEG; Sigma—melted, neutralized, and pre-warmed to 37 °C).

1 N HCL.

pH test paper.

Disposable sterile 0.22-μm syringe filter.

Iscove's medium with L-glutamine and sodium bicarbonate (3.024 g/L).

Iscove's medium with 10 % FBS.

HAT-selective medium; Iscove's with 10 % FBS and 1× HAT from 100× stock supplemented with 10 % macrophage-conditioned medium (MCM) (*see* **Note** 7).

HT-selective medium; Iscove's with 10 % FBS and 1× HT from 50× stock.

---

3   Methods

3.1 Preparation of Cell Culture Medium

We prefer to use dry-powered Iscove's versus premade liquid medium as it has better storage and shelf life. This dry formulation contains L-glutamine but requires the addition of 3.024 g/L of sodium bicarbonate. Medium is dissolved in ultrapure water and bicarbonate added (shift in yellow solution to red). From this stock Iscove's solution, three medium formulations are made: (1) Iscove's with 10 % fetal bovine serum (FBS), (2) Iscove's with 10 % FBS and 10 % macrophage-conditioned media (MCM) and 1 × HAT from 100 × HAT stock, and (3) Iscove's with 10 % FBS and 1 × HT from 50 × HT stock. All solutions are sterile filtered into sterile media bottles (*see* **Note** 8).

3.2 Preparation of Solid PEG (Polyethylene Glycol)

Place a 5-g bottle of PEG (Sigma P2906; 3,000–3,700 MW) on a hot plate to liquefy the wax. One must monitor this so as not to overheat the PEG. Place a needle through the membrane as a pressure release device so the top won't pop off. Use "high heat" setting and monitor the melt which should yield ~4 mL. Once liquefied, add 5 mL of stock Iscove's (*no serum*) and then add 700 μl of DMSO (Sigma D2650; 5-mL bottle) followed by 1–2 drops of 1 N HCL until slightly acidic/neutral pH is achieved—test using pH strip paper. Filter sterilize the ~10 mL PEG through a 0.22-μm syringe filter into a sterile tube and place in 37 °C water bath until needed.

3.3 Preparation of Splenocytes

Immunized mice are anesthetized then euthanized by cervical dislocation and placed in a laminar hood, body saturated in 70 % alcohol, and spleens aseptically removed (trim clean) and placed in a tube containing 25 mL of sterile pre-warmed 37 °C Iscove's medium with 10 % FBS. Perform one fusion at a time at a steady pace. Open a sterile 100 mm Petrie dish and place the sterile stainless steel sieve with mesh on the bottom of the dish. Pour the spleen and medium into the sieve then using a sterile glass pestle or sterile plunger from a 5 mL syringe mash the spleen through the metal mesh of the sieve toward the bottom of the Petri dish to obtain a cell suspension. Using a sterile pipette, pass and mash fresh media through ~10 mL through the sieve to dislodge and push through cells; leave any fatty connective tissue on the mesh screen. Remove sieve and transfer the dispersed cells in media from the bottom of the dish through a 100 μm sterile nylon cell strainer into a fresh 50 mL sterile conical tube. Add fresh media slowly to the cell strainer and gently mash bits with a sterile 5 mL syringe plunger through the nylon mesh to pass and transfer cell suspension into tube. Centrifuge cells at 1,500 rpm for 5 min in a swinging bucket clinical centrifuge to pellet, aspirate and discard supernatant then gently suspend cell pellet in 10 mL of pre-warmed red cell lysis buffer and incubate for 10 min at 37 °C; at this time begin preparation of myeloma cells. After 10 min incubation in RBC lysis buffer centrifuge splenocytes to pellet and resuspend in Iscove's medium *without FBS*. Count cells to determine yield (we routinely recover ~ 10^8 splenocytes).

3.4 Preparation of Myeloma Cells

Myeloma cells grow in suspension forming cell clusters. We use several large flasks to maintain cells for harvest and 1 day before fusion cells are subcultured into fresh media to maximize growth and health. To harvest myeloma cells from culture flasks we gently scrape the flask bottom and transfer the cell suspension into a 50 mL conical tube, centrifuge at 1,500 rpm for 5 min in clinical centrifuge to pellet, aspirate the media and suspend the cells in pre-warmed Iscove's basal medium without FBS and repeat centrifugation. Finally we suspend the cells in fresh Iscove's without FBS and count cells to determine yield (*see* **Note 9**).

3.5 Performing Myeloma-Splenocyte Cell Fusion

1. One day prior to cell fusion subclone growing myeloma cells.

2. On day of fusion prepare PEG solution.

3. Sacrifice immunized mouse, aseptically harvest spleen and prepare splenocytes for cell fusion.

4. Prepare myeloma cells for cell fusion.

5. Combine myeloma and splenocyte cell suspensions (Iscove's without FBS) to achieve a splenocyte to myeloma ratio of 1:1 in a fresh sterile 50 mL conical tube, swirl and invert tube, centrifuge at 1,500 rpm for 5 min to pellet and aspirate medium (*see* **Note 10**).

6. Place a small beaker half-filled with pre-warmed 37 °C water in the laminar flow hood or small heater block that will hold a 50 mL tube.

7. Tap the tube bottom containing the combined splenocytes and myeloma cell pellet on the bottom of the bench several times to loosen the packed cell pellet. Keep cells in tube warm by using the water filled beaker.

8. Transfer 1 mL of pre-warmed stock PEG solution into a sterile 1.5 mL microcentrifuge tube. Transfer 2 mL and 7 mL of pre-warmed Iscove's medium without serum into two sterile tubes and keep in water bath.

9. To the tube containing the cell pellet, slowly add 1 mL of PEG dropwise at a rate over 1 min using a Pasteur pipette with a dispensing bulb to the top of cell pellet maintained in the beaker water bath while gently rocking the tube containing cells. Using the tip of the Pasteur pipette, gently mix cells and the viscous PEG. Repeat this process until the entire 1 mL of PEG is dispensed in the tube with the cells. Allow the cells to rest in PEG for 30–90 s.

10. Add 2 mL of Iscove's medium without serum dropwise using a Pasteur pipette at a rate over 2 min while rocking the tube with cells gently to slowly dilute the PEG concentration over time.

11. Add 7 mL Iscove's medium without serum dropwise using a Pasteur pipette at a rate over 5 min while rocking the tube with cells gently to further dilute the PEG concentration over time.

12. The newly fused cells are fragile at this point, be gentle!

13. Using an Erlenmeyer flask add Iscove's HAT medium to approximate the volume × microplate number that you want to spread the cells over. Generally we will do 10 × 96-well microtiter plates per fusion at 200 μL/well; so ~200 mL of HAT medium is added into the flask. Pour in the fused cells from the tube into HAT media contained in the flask; use a small volume of medium to rinse the residual from the tube. Gently swirl the mixture to disperse the cells evenly. Pour cell suspension from flask into large sterile solution basin ~50–100 mL at a time for cell plating. Using a multichannel pipette transfer 200 μL of cell suspension into each well of 10 microliter cell culture plates and move plates to CO_2 incubator (*see* **Note 11**).

14. Hybridoma colonies should begin to form in 7–10 days. We usually use one plate from the fusion to evaluate efficiency by counting the total number of wells with at least one colony. Most wells will have a significant amount of debris but live cell colonies should be obvious using a phase contrast microscope as shown in Fig. 2. Wells with growing cells will start to yellow as they become more acidic and the culture medium has a finite limit. Accumulation of mAb is progressive in the medium so swapping medium requires time to renew the mAb concentration. The decision on when to screen plates will depend on the size of the colonies; too early and there is not enough mAb produced to yield a good signal; too late and colonies are large making isolation of single cell clones producing mAb more difficult.

15. The strategy for screening hybridoma wells was discussed in the introduction. We screen full plates by ELISA and do not screen for colonies. This facilitates automation via plate washing and reading; it also provides a strong baseline background measure for the assay. We usually use 75–100 μL of the culture supernatant transferred aseptically to prepped non-sterile high-binding ELISA plates using a multichannel pipette (*see* **Note 12**). The ELISA is usually completed within the same day and results evaluated. Obvious positives wells are identified and less obvious positives are compared to background established from the entire ten plates. Positive hits by ELISA are then identified by location on the culture plates and the presence of hybridoma in those wells deemed as positive microscopically. It is not unusual to find strong positive wells without cells; this likely reflects antibody produced by hybridoma that failed to survive, e.g., unstable hybridoma, or production from a primary cell that has died.

16. Cells from positive mAb producing wells determined by the primary screen are transferred using a P1000 tip to a 48-well culture plate containing Iscove's HT medium and allowed to grow on 3–4 days. If the original 96-well cell colony is small those may be allowed to grow additional time to achieve a reasonable cell density prior to transfer to the larger 24-well plate. Cells that survive this transfer are evaluated in a secondary screen by ELISA titration of culture supernatant. The secondary screen is highly useful as it allows for a more rational decision concerning which cell to clone. Each 24-well contains ~1 mL of hybridoma supernatant so multiple ELISA's, Western blots, and titrations can be performed to address specificity and sensitivity. Those cell/wells that titrate activity are then isolated by limiting dilution back on 96-well plates in HT medium; allowed to grow and evaluated by screening the wells. Limiting dilution is performed until you are confident the cells are cloned at which time they are further expanded in Iscove's/FBS and frozen vials stored. At this time cloned cells can be used to make ascites and/or cell conditioned media used for mAb characterization.

4   Notes

1. Small peptide or haptens often bind poorly to microtiter screening plates used in ELISA and the addition of a large protein carrier serves to facilitate binding to plastic and orients the molecule for antibody binding.

2. During hybridoma screening those that produce IgM antibodies can be problematic as they tend to be "sticky" and given their multi-unit properties generate huge signals with secondary

antibody reporters. In our experience these tend to be nonspecific false positives, and we avoid IgM detection by using isotype-specific secondary antibody reporters.

3. Polyclonal anti-sera often provide the best choice when trying to identify an in-solution capture capable mAb. Here a non-murine species is best to minimize unwanted binding and high background due to insufficient blocking of the anti-mouse mAb used to capture the hybridoma supernatant. Although direct binding of the hybridoma supernatant to the microassay plate can be done, often there is limited mAb produced at this stage of hybridoma screening and lots of cell culture media proteins that serve to limit binding of mAb to the plate in sufficient quantities to evoke a strong reporter signal.

4. We use submandibular "cheek" puncture to harvest ~200 μL of blood into a 1.5 mL microcentrifuge tube [8]. After coagulation we spin down the cells and harvest the sera. Log dilutions of the polyclonal anti-sera are then evaluated for antigen binding per the defined ELISA screening strategy. Western "slot blots" can also be performed to evaluate molecular weight of protein targets to increase confidence of immunogenicity. If sera have a low antibody titer, those animals can be boosted again with immunogen and anti-sera harvested a second time. In general there should be 10+ days between immunogen/adjuvant boosts and anti-sera harvested 10–14 days after the final adjuvant boost to yield maximal antibody titer.

5. The non-adjuvant intraperitoneal (i.p.) boost 3 days prior to cell fusion is thought to facilitate mobilization and expansion of antibody producing plasma and B-cells to the spleen and thereby maximize the potential for hybrid formation to the desired cell type.

6. Myeloma cells should be occasionally re-cloned from a single cell, evaluated for IgG production (negative), and challenged with 6-thioguanine (6-TG) or 8-azaguanine to validate HGPRT deficiency.

7. Although not essential, macrophage-conditioned medium (MCM) can provide additional growth factors that improve the chance of hybridoma survival. MCM is produced by growing 1×10^6 J774.2 macrophage-like cells in cell culture flasks (T75) overnight (Iscove's with 10 % FBS) and harvesting supernatant; this process can be repeated after scraping cells and re-seeding flasks. The resulting MCM is centrifuged and sterile filtered to remove cells and debris. MCM can be stored frozen until needed and is used at 5–20 % to supplement HAT medium.

8. Fetal bovine serum (FBS) varies and each batch should be evaluated for cell support before purchase; switching between lots of FBS is not advised and all cell culture performed should be

maintained in the same lot of FBS. FBS should be thawed at 4 °C and can be stored at this temperature sterile for several months. We also prefer to use heat-inactivated FBS for our cell culture to minimize unwanted active proteins in the medium; this can be purchased from vendors or heat inactivation can be performed precisely by holding FBS at 56 °C for 30 min. Aminopterin is light sensitive and HAT medium should be protected from light.

9. Proteins are precipitated by PEG and fusion efficiency will be poor with residual protein like FBS, so wash cells to remove FBS proteins prior to the fusion step.

10. The ratio of splenocyte to myeloma can be varied and improved efficiencies might be achieved by changing the cell ratios. The cell fusion is a random process and the goal is to maximize splenocyte-myeloma fusion events.

11. We usually evaluate the first plate for cell density and determine if further dilution is necessary. Remember the vast majority of cells will not survive. Fused cell suspension can be plated over any number of culture plates. As more microtiter plates are used per fusion the lower the initial cell density per well. This can be beneficial to subsequent cell cloning where optimal conditions would be a single growing hybridoma clone per well. In some cases we have plated the fused cells over 100×96-well microtiter plates. The decision on plate number is a balance of cost to benefit. Wells with positives assay activity and more than one hybridoma colony require cloning to identify and isolate the cell producing the mAb of interest. In general we might expect to see between 40 and 70 % fusion efficiency with those wells having 1–4 hybridoma colonies.

12. The transfer of sterile culture supernatant into a non-sterile ELISA plate should be done with care to avoid introducing contamination. This process requires a significant number of P200 tips. Often we use one set of tips per plate accepting some well-to-well mAb cross over that might skew our screening data; this must be done carefully to avoid touching tips to non-sterile plates. Alternatively one can use a Transtar system from Costar that uses 96-tip cartridges to do the transfer in bulk from each plate.

References

1. Kohler G, Milstein C (1975) Continuous cultures of fused cells secreting antibody of predefined specificity. Nature 256:495–497

2. Kohler G, Howe SC, Milstein C (1976) Fusion between immunoglobulin-secreting and nonsecreting myeloma cell lines. Eur J Immunol 6:292–295

3. Galfre G, Howe SC, Milstein C et al (1977) Antibodies to major histocompatibility antigens produced by hybrid cell lines. Nature 266:550–552

4. Shulman M, Wilde CD, Kohler G (1978) A better cell line for making hybridomas secreting specific antibodies. Nature 276:269–270

5. Galfre G, Milstein C (1981) Preparation of monolconal antibodies: strategies and procedures. Methods Enzymol 73B:3–46

6. Hurrell JGR (1982) Monoclonal hybridoma antibodies: techniques and applications. CRC Press, Boca Raton, FL

7. Schreier M, Kohler G, Hengartner H et al (1980) Hybridoma Techniques: EMBO, SKMB Course 1980, Basel. Cold Spring Harbor, New York

8. Golde WT, Gollobin P, Rodriguez LL (2005) A rapid, simple, and humane method for submandibular bleeding of mice using a lancet. Lab Anim 9:39–43

Chapter 3

Affinity Purification of Antibodies

Robert M. Hnasko and Jeffery A. McGarvey

Abstract

Antibodies are provided in a variety of formats that include antiserum, hybridoma culture supernatant, or ascites. They can all be used successfully in crude form for the detection of target antigens by immunoassay. However, it is advantageous to use purified antibody in defined quantity to facilitate assay reproducibility, economy, and reduced interference of nonspecific components as well as improved storage, stability, and bio-conjugation. Although not always necessary, the relative simplicity of antibody purification using commercially available protein-A, protein-G, or protein-L resins with basic chromatographic principles warrants purification when antibody source material is available in sufficient quantity. Here, we define three simple methods using immobilized (1) protein-A, (2) protein-G, and (3) protein-L agarose beads to yield highly purified antibody.

Key words Antibody, Ascites, Antiserum, Hybridoma-conditioned medium, Affinity purification, Protein-A, Protein-G, Protein-L, Liquid chromatography

1 Introduction

A variety of methods are available for the purification of antibodies, and the choice depends on the intended application, the species of origin, immunoglobulin (Ig) class and subclass, and the source of starting material. It is important to recognize that no single method can fulfill the requirements for all application needs, but those detailed in this chapter provide common methods suitable for most IgG purification. To maximize IgG purification, we take advantage of high-capacity IgG binding by specific bacterial proteins immobilized on a solid support such as agarose or Sepharose beads. The bacterial proteins used in the purification of antibodies are (1) protein-A derived from *Staphylococcus aureus*, (2) protein-G from *Streptococcus* sp., and (3) protein-L from *Peptostreptococcus magnus* [1–4]. Each of these proteins provides unique Ig-binding properties, outlined in Table 1, which can be used for purification of antibodies from a variety of matrices such as serum, culture supernatant, or ascites [5, 6].

Robert Hnasko (ed.), *ELISA: Methods and Protocols*, Methods in Molecular Biology, vol. 1318,
DOI 10.1007/978-1-4939-2742-5_3, © Springer Science+Business Media New York 2015

Table 1
Antibody binding properties of bacterial protein-A, protein-G, and protein-L

	Native protein-A	Recombinant protein-A	Native protein-G	Recombinant protein-G	Recombinant protein-A/protein-G	Recombinant protein-L
Native source	*Staphylococcus aureus*	*Staphylococcus aureus*	*G. Streptococcus* sp. *C. Streptococcus* sp.	*Streptococcus* sp.	*Staphylococcus aureus* *Streptococcus* sp.	*Peptostreptococcus magnus*
MW (Da)	46,700	44,600	65,000 G148 protein-G 40,000 G43 protein-G 58,000 C40 protein-G	21,600	50,460	35,800
# Ig-binding sites	5	5	2	2	4 + 2	4
Ig-binding target	Fc	Fc	Fc, Fab	Fc	Fc	VL-kappa
Albumin-binding site	No	No	Yes G148 and C40 No G43	No	No	No
Optimal binding pH	8.2	8.2	5	5	5–8.2	7.5

Protein-A and protein-G have binding sites for the Fc portion of mammalian antibodies. Native protein-G contains binding sites for Fab region of antibodies as well as albumin. Recombinant protein-G has been engineered to eliminate Fab and albumin binding. Protein-L binding is limited to specific subclasses of the kappa light chain. Protein-L does not bind to bovine, ovine, or donkey as their antibodies are composed almost exclusively of lambda light chains; it will bind to chicken IgY

Polyclonal antibodies are frequently provided as an antiserum obtained from blood of immunized animals. Raw antiserum contains a large number of extraneous proteins that can interfere with immunoassays, and protein-A or protein-G is commonly used to eliminate the bulk of unwanted serum proteins. Antisera also contain a large number of unwanted antibodies (>95 % total IgG) against non-antigen targets, and these nonspecific Ig proteins are not removed by this purification method. Monoclonal antibodies are often provided as a hybridoma culture supernatant or as ascitic fluid harvested from the intraperitoneal cavity of mice after inoculation with a clonal hybridoma cell line. Similar to polyclonal antisera, monoclonal antibodies can be purified by protein-A or protein-G methods, but unlike antisera, the majority of immunoglobulins present in the crude fluid are of a singular class/subtype directed against the target antigen [7, 8]. Protein-L can often be substituted for protein-A or protein-G, and we take advantage of its inability to bind bovine IgG to purify mouse IgG from hybridoma culture supernatant, which is supplemented with fetal bovine serum (FBS). The relative binding affinities of these three antibody-binding proteins for IgG types from different species are provided in Table 2. Neither protein-A nor protein-G bind IgY antibodies derived from chicken egg so purification is limited to protein-L. The typical concentration of antibody in antiserum is 1–3 mg/mL; hybridoma culture supernatant is 0.1–10 mg/mL and ascites 2–10 mg/mL as shown in Table 3 [6]. Prior to purification, crude antisera and ascites should be diluted in appropriate buffer to adjust binding pH and minimize bulk protein load effects that can block desired antibody binding to the resin.

2 Materials

Disposable column capable of containing at least 2 mL resin bed volume.

Immobilized protein-A, protein-G, or protein-L agarose/ Sepharose beads (*see* **Note 1**).

Liquid chromatography system as shown in Fig. 1 or handheld syringe-column system as shown in Fig. 2.

Antisera, ascites, or hybridoma culture supernatant.

Centrifuge.

Disposable centrifuge tubes (1.5–50 mL).

Disposable transfer pipette or syringe.

0.2 μm filter.

1 N HCl.

1 N NaOH.

Table 2
Relative binding affinities of antibodies from different species to protein-A, protein-G, and protein-L

Species	Ig Class	Protein-A	Protein-G	Protein-L (κ) light chains only
Mouse	Total IgG	++++	++++	++++
	IgG1	+	++++	++++
	IgG2a	++++	++++	++++
	IgG2b	+++	+++	++++
	IgG3	++	+++	++++
Human	Total IgG	++++	++++	++++
	IgG1	++++	++++	++++
	IgG2	++++	++++	++++
	IgG3	+	++++	++++
	IgG4	++++	++++	++++
	IgA	–	–	++++
	IgD	–	–	++++
	IgE	–	–	++++
	IgM	–	–	++++
	κ	–	–	++++
	λ	–	–	–
	Fab	++	++	++++
	scFv	++	–	++++
Rat	Total IgG	+	+	++++
	IgG1	–	+	++++
	IgG2a	–	++++	++++
	IgG2b	–	++	++++
	IgG2c	+	++	++++
Rabbit	Total IgG	++++	+++	+
Donkey	Total IgG	++	++++	–
Sheep	Total IgG	+	++	–
	IgG1	+	++	–
	IgG2	+++	+++	–
Goat	Total IgG	+	++	–
	IgG1	+	+++	–
	IgG2	+++	+++	–
Cow	Total IgG	++	++++	–
	IgG1	+	+++	–
	IgG2	+++	+++	–
Chicken	Total IgG	–	+	++

Thimerosal.

pH meter.

UV monitor for protein absorbance at 280 nm or protein assay such as Bradford or bicinchoninic acid (BCA).

Protein-A binding buffer: 0.1 M phosphate buffer, 0.15 M sodium chloride; pH 8.0.

Table 3
Concentration of antibody and major contaminating proteins found in serum, hybridoma supernatant, ascitic fluid, and egg yolk

Source	Immunoglobulins	Contaminants	Quantity (mg/mL)
Mouse serum	Polyclonal	Albumin, transferrin, alpha-2-macroglobulin	IgG 2–5 mg/mL IgM 0.8–7 mg/mL IgA 1–3 mg/mL
Hybridoma-conditioned medium (10 % FBS)	Monoclonal	Phenol red, water, albumin, transferrin, bovine IgG	0.01–1 mg/mL
Ascitic fluid	Monoclonal	Lipids, albumin, transferrin, lipoproteins, endogenous IgG	0.5–10 mg/mL
Egg yolk	IgY	Lipids, lipoproteins	3–4 mg/mL

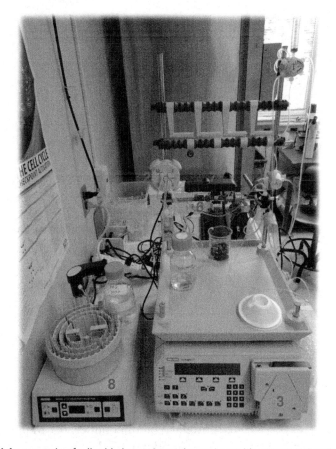

Fig. 1 An example of a liquid chromatography system with component parts and liquid plumbing. (*1*) Liquid chromatography controller; (*2*) buffer selection valve; (*3*) peristaltic pump; (*4*) sample loop; (*5*) diverter valve; (*6*) column holder; (*7*) UV monitor (280 nm); (*8*) fraction collector

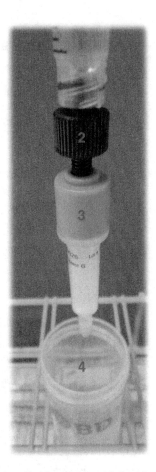

Fig. 2 An example of a handheld manual push liquid chromatography system. (*1*) Female thread Luer-lock syringe; (*2*) black syringe attachment nut with male Luer-lock end and column thread; (*3*) 1 mL protein-G packed column with female thread input for syringe attachment nut and male thread output opening; (*4*) collection tube

Protein-A elution buffers: 0.1 M citric acid (pH 3.0–6.5).

    pH 6.5 for IgG1.

    pH 4.5 for IgG2a and IgG2b.

    pH 3.0 for IgG3.

Protein-G binding buffer: sodium acetate (pH 5.0).

Protein-G and protein-L elution buffer: 0.1 M glycine-HCL (pH 2–3).

Protein-L binding buffer: 0.1 M phosphate buffer, 0.15 M sodium chloride; pH 7.2.

Neutralization buffer: high-ionic strength alkaline buffer such as 1 M phosphate or 1 M Tris (pH 7.5–9).

Dialysis bag/cassette or desalting column for buffer exchange.

Storage buffer: 30 % ethanol in water or 0.05 % thimerosal in water.

3   Methods

3.1   Antibody Purification Using Immobilized Protein-A

1. Protein-A purification is recommended for human IgG, and antibody is bound at slightly basic pH and eluted at an acidic pH (*see* **Note 2**).

2. Equilibrate the protein-A agarose and reagents to room temperature before use.

3. Clarify antibody fluids (antisera, ascites, or hybridoma supernatant) by centrifugation at $20,000 \times g$ for 20 min at 4 °C or room temperature and collect supernatant (*see* **Note 3**).

4. Adjust pH of sample by dilution of antisera or ascitic fluid 1:10 with protein-A binding buffer (pH 8.0) or 1:2 for hybridoma cell-conditioned medium with 1 N NaOH used to adjust pH to 8.0 as necessary. Save a small volume fraction and label as input.

5. Prepare protein-A column by washing with 3–5× column volumes of binding buffer at 1 mL/min to remove preservative and exchange buffer and pH.

6. Pass clarified antibody sample in binding buffer over column 1–3× at a rate of 0.5–1 mL/min (*see* **Note 4**). Monitor protein absorbance at 280 nm using an in-line UV monitor as shown in Fig. 1 (*see* **Note 5**). Save a small volume of the sample after it has been passed over the column and label as unbound (*see* **Note 6**).

7. Pass at least 5× column volume of protein-A binding buffer at 1 mL/min to wash beads of residual unbound protein and return to baseline 280 nm absorbance values. Save a small volume from each column pass of wash buffer and label them as wash 1–5 (*see* **Note 7**).

8. Apply protein-A elution buffer at a rate of 1 mL/min and begin collecting 1 mL fractions after approximately 1× column volume (*see* **Note 8**). Collect 1 mL fractions into tubes containing 0.1 mL of 1 M neutralization buffer (PBS; pH 8) to immediately neutralize acidic pH of the elution fraction. Monitor protein absorbance at 280 nm UV to identify desorption of the IgG from the resin as an A_{280} protein peak and collect fractions until baseline protein measurement is achieved (*see* **Note 9**). Save a small volume from each elution fraction and label them as elution 1–5.

9. Determine protein concentration of each fraction by measuring absorbance at 280 nm or performing a protein assay such as Bradford or BCA. Plot the protein concentration of each fraction and evaluate the protein profile from all the fractions to identify those containing the antibody and ensure proper column performance. An example of an antibody elution profile is shown in Fig. 3 (*see* **Note 10**).

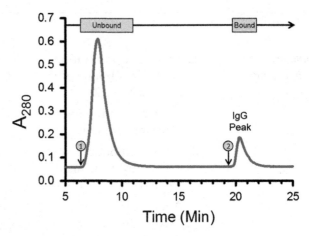

Fig. 3 A representative protein absorbance profile (A_{280} nm) following protein-G affinity purification (1 mL column) of monoclonal antibody from ascites at 1 mL/min. Column equilibration was performed with binding buffer alone resulting in a stable baseline absorbance (1–6 min). Ascites was added beginning at ①, and a large protein absorbance peak was measured between 7 and 10 min showing the unbound protein that does not bind protein-G resin. The ascites were followed by wash buffer alone until a stable background absorbance was reestablished between 11 and 19 min. Elution buffer was added at ② resulting in elution of an IgG protein peak between 20 and 22 min with a return to baseline absorbance observed at 24 min

10. Pool and dialyze peak antibody fractions using a low molecular weight cutoff membrane against desired buffer such as PBS. Collect purified and desalted antibody for downstream application (*see* **Note 11**).

11. Regenerate the affinity resin by washing with 5× column volume of binding buffer followed by 5× column elution buffer [9] (*see* **Note 12**).

12. To store the column, pass 5× column volumes of storage buffer that contains a bacteriostatic agent such as 0.05 % thimerosal or 30 % ethanol solution in water (*see* **Note 13**). Keep excess solution in the column to maintain resin hydration and store capped at 4 °C.

3.2 Antibody Purification Using Immobilized Protein-G

1. Protein-G purification is recommended for mouse IgG, and antibody is bound at slightly acidic pH and eluted at a more acidic pH.

2. Equilibrate the protein-G agarose and reagents to room temperature before use.

3. Clarify antibody fluids (antisera, ascites, or hybridoma supernatant) by centrifugation at 20,000×*g* for 20 min at 4 °C or room temperature and collect supernatant (*see* **Note 3**).

4. Adjust pH of sample by dilution of antisera or ascitic fluid 1:10 with protein-G binding buffer (0.1 M sodium acetate; pH 5.0) or 1:2 for hybridoma-conditioned medium. Save small volume of sample and label input.

5. Prepare protein-G column by washing with 3–5× column volumes of protein-G binding buffer at a rate of 1 mL/min to remove preservative and exchange buffer and pH.

6. Pass clarified antibody sample in binding buffer over column 1–3× at a rate of 0.5–1 mL/min (*see* **Note 4**). Monitor protein absorbance at 280 nm using an in-line UV monitor as shown in Fig. 1 (*see* **Note 5**). Save a small volume of the sample after it has been passed over the column and label as unbound (*see* **Note 6**).

7. Pass at least 5× column volume of protein-G binding buffer at 1 mL/min to wash beads of residual unbound protein and return to baseline 280 nm absorbance values. Save a small volume from each column pass of wash buffer and label them as wash 1–5 (*see* **Note 7**).

8. Apply protein-G elution buffer (0.1 M glycine-HCL, pH 2–3) at a rate of 1 mL/min and begin collecting 1 mL fractions into tube containing 0.1 mL of neutralization buffer (1 M Tris buffer, pH 8.0). Monitor protein absorbance at 280 nm UV to identify desorption of the IgG from the resin as an A_{280} protein peak and collect fractions until baseline protein measurement is achieved (*see* **Note 9**). Save a small volume from each elution fraction and label them as elution 1–5.

9. Determine protein concentration of each fraction by measuring absorbance at 280 nm or performing a protein assay such as Bradford or BCA. Plot the protein concentration of each fraction and evaluate the protein profile from all the fractions to identify those containing the antibody and ensure proper column performance. An example of an antibody elution profile is shown in Fig. 3 (*see* **Note 10**).

10. Pool and dialyze peak antibody fractions using a low molecular weight cutoff membrane against desired buffer such as PBS. Collect purified and desalted antibody for downstream application (*see* **Note 11**).

11. Regenerate the affinity resin by washing with 5× column volume of binding buffer followed by 5× column elution buffer [9] (*see* **Note 12**).

12. To store the column, pass 5× column volumes of storage buffer that contains a bacteriostatic agent such as 0.05 % thimerosal or 30 % ethanol solution in water (*see* **Note 13**). Keep excess solution in the column to maintain resin hydration and store capped at 4 °C.

3.3 Immobilized Protein-L

1. Protein-L purification is recommended for hybridoma cell-conditioned medium containing fetal bovine serum, and antibody is bound at neutral pH and eluted at an acidic pH (*see* **Note 14**).

2. Equilibrate the protein-L agarose and reagents to room temperature before use.

3. Centrifuge hybridoma supernatant to remove cells and debris at $10,000 \times g$ for 5 min at room temperature then pass supernatant through a 0.2 μm filter.

4. Dilute sample at least 1:1 with protein-L binding buffer (PB, pH 7.2) before applying onto the protein-L column to maintain optimal ionic strength and pH for binding. Save a small volume of fraction and label as input.

5. Prepare protein-L column by washing with 3–5× column volumes of protein-L binding buffer at a rate of 1 mL/min to remove preservative and exchange buffer and pH.

6. Pass clarified antibody sample in binding buffer over column 1–3× at a rate of 0.5–1 mL/min (*see* **Note 4**). Monitor protein absorbance at 280 nm using an in-line UV monitor as shown in Fig. 1 (*see* **Note 5**). Save a small volume of the sample after it has been passed over the column and label as unbound (*see* **Note 6**).

7. Pass at least 5× column volume of protein-L binding buffer at 1 mL/min to wash beads of residual unbound protein and return to baseline 280 nm absorbance values. Save a small volume from each column pass of wash buffer and label them as wash 1–5 (*see* **Note 7**).

8. Apply protein-L elution buffer (0.1 M glycine-HCL, pH 2–3) at a rate of 1 mL/min and begin collecting 1 mL fractions into tube containing 0.1 mL of neutralization buffer (1 M Tris buffer, pH 8.0). Monitor protein absorbance at 280 nm UV to identify desorption of the IgG from the resin as an A_{280} protein peak and collect fractions until baseline protein measurement is achieved (*see* **Note 9**). Save a small volume from each elution fraction and label them as elution 1–5.

9. Determine protein concentration of each fraction by measuring absorbance at 280 nm or performing a protein assay such as Bradford or BCA. Plot the protein concentration of each fraction and evaluate the protein profile from all the fractions to identify those containing the antibody and ensure proper column performance. An example of an antibody elution profile is shown in Fig. 3 (*see* **Note 10**).

10. Pool and dialyze peak antibody fractions using a low molecular weight cutoff membrane against desired buffer such as PBS.

Collect purified and desalted antibody for downstream application (*see* **Note 11**).

11. Regenerate the affinity resin by washing with 5× column volume of binding buffer followed by 5× column elution buffer [9] (*see* **Note 12**).

12. To store the column, pass 5× column volumes of storage buffer that contains a bacteriostatic agent such as 0.05 % thimerosal or 30 % ethanol solution in water (*see* **Note 13**). Keep excess solution in the column to maintain resin hydration and store capped at 4 °C.

4 Notes

1. Do not freeze or vortex agarose beads. Gently invert or swirl to mix beads; this avoids strong shear forces that will damage and fragment the beads that negatively impact performance.

2. Sample pH of 8.0 is optimal for binding of IgG1, whereas other Ig subclasses bind better at pH 7.4.

3. Centrifugation is used to remove solids that can block column flow. Harvest supernatants and discard debris. Filtration can be used as an alternative or additional step with 0.2 μm sufficient for sterility. Ascitic fluid will contain lipids and should be first passed through a small amount of glass wool to bind fats and lipids. Squeeze the fluid from the glass wool to harvest antibody containing liquid to be centrifuged. Discard the glass wool bundle.

4. Passing fluid over a column can be accomplished by either gravity flow, manually pushing fluid by way of Luer-lock syringe, or peristaltic pump. The column bed volume (volume of resin) and antibody binding capacity should be determined based on the volume and protein concentration of the sample. High protein loads will interfere with specific binding, and sample dilution is used to reduce potential bulk protein load interference. The flow rate and pressure also affect binding and should be maintained within manufacture specifications of the column.

5. In-line monitoring of 280 nm absorbance is a convenient way of monitoring protein concentration in real time. This provides a rapid assessment of column performance and antibody elution without the need for downstream evaluation of individual fractions. If this is not available, measuring the protein concentration of each individual labeled fraction can provide the evaluation at the end of the run. Estimate of IgG concentration based on 280 nm absorbance; $1.43\ A_{280} = 1$ mg/mL.

6. If the sample contains an antibody type that does not bind to the affinity resin or exceeds the binding capacity, the flow-through will contain excess antibody, and the unbound antibody can be recovered and examined by antibody-specific assays. Optimally, the unbound material will not contain any desired antibody.

7. The last wash fractions should have 280 nm absorbance values similar to binding buffer alone.

8. The optimal pH of protein-A elution buffers composed of 0.1 M citric acid may vary for antibody isotype from pH 3.0 for IgG3, pH 4.5 for IgG2a and IgG2b, and pH 6.5 for IgG1.

9. An alternative to collecting individual elution fractions, one can collect a single tube of the entire IgG peak. This can be accomplished by monitoring the A_{280} and collecting just the volume associated with the IgG protein peak. This can maximize antibody concentration by reducing total volume.

10. Evaluate antibody-antigen binding and IgG profile from column fractions to determine if the affinity chromatography conditions are suitable for purification and adjust binding buffer or elution buffer pH as necessary. If binding to protein-A is ineffective, switch to alternate protein-G or protein-L resins and associated methodologies.

11. Avoid dialysis against amine-based buffers such as Tris as these often interfere with downstream labeling reactions. One way to increase antibody concentration is using centrifuge concentrators with low molecular weight cutoff membranes to reduce volume.

12. Regeneration of binding resin using a stronger acidified elution buffer can aid in removing any residual antibody or binding of unwanted protein. Columns can be regenerated multiple times and used to purify the same or different antibodies.

13. Avoid the use of sodium azide as it represents a disposal hazard and is incompatible with horseradish peroxidase-labeled antibodies.

14. Protein-L does not bind bovine antibodies. This is relevant when purification is done from hybridoma-conditioned medium that contains fetal bovine serum (FBS).

References

1. Goding JW (1978) Use of staphylococcal protein A as an immunological reagent. J Immunol Methods 20:241–253

2. Akerström B, Björck LJ (1989) Protein L: an immunoglobulin light chain-binding bacterial protein. Characterization of binding and physicochemical properties. J Biol Chem 264: 19740–19746

3. Housden NG, Harrison S, Roberts SE et al (2003) Immunoglobulin-binding domains: protein L from Peptostreptococcus magnus. Biochem Soc Trans 31:716–718

4. Vola R, Lombardi A, Tarditi L et al (1995) Recombinant proteins L and LG: efficient tools for purification of murine immunoglobulin G fragments. J Chromatogr B Biomed Appl 668:209–218

5. Tashiro M, Montelione GT (1995) Structures of bacterial immunoglobulin-binding domains and their complexes with immunoglobulins. Curr Opin Struct Biol 5:471–481

6. Lindmark R, Thorén-Tolling K, Sjöquist J (1983) Binding of immunoglobulins to protein A and immunoglobulin levels in mammalian sera. J Immunol Methods 62:1–13

7. Huse K, Böhme HJ, Scholz GH (2002) Purification of antibodies by affinity chromatography. J Biochem Biophys Methods 51:217–231

8. Ayyar BV, Arora S, Murphy C et al (2012) Affinity chromatography as a tool for antibody purification. Methods 56:116–129

9. Bill E, Lutz U, Karlsson BM et al (1995) Optimization of protein G chromatography for biopharmaceutical monoclonal antibodies. J Mol Recognit 8:90–94

Chapter 4

Bioconjugation of Antibodies to Horseradish Peroxidase (HRP)

Robert M. Hnasko

Abstract

The bioconjugation of an antibody to an enzymatic reporter such as horseradish peroxidase (HRP) affords an effective mechanism by which immunoassay detection of a target antigen can be achieved. The use of heterobifunctional cross-linkers to covalently link antibodies to HRP provides a simple and convenient means to maintain antibody affinity while imparting a functional reporter used for antigen detection. In this chapter, we describe a process by which Sulfo-SMCC is used to generate a stable maleimide-activated HRP that is reactive with sulfhydryl groups generated in antibodies by SATA-mediated thiolation.

Key words Bioconjugation, Heterobifunctional cross-linker, Antibody, Horseradish peroxidase (HRP), SMCC, SATA, Maleimide, Thiolation

1 Introduction

Horseradish peroxidase (HRP) is a 40,000 Da enzyme that can catalyze the reaction of hydrogen peroxide with an organic electron-donating substrate to form a color, fluorescent, or chemiluminescent product upon oxidation [1, 2]. The use of antibody-HRP or streptavidin-HRP bioconjugates as part of an enhanced chemiluminescent (ECL) assay provides an extremely sensitive reporter for the detection of target antigen by ELISA and Western blotting applications [3].

The relatively small size of HRP facilitates access to antigenic sites or structures in the target antigen. Moreover, the enzyme remains stable and functional under multiple conditions that include chemical cross-linking, freeze drying, or prolonged storage at 4 °C.

HRP is a glycoprotein, and its polysaccharide chains are often used in cross-linking reactions to couple the enzyme to an antibody. Mild oxidation of sugars with sodium periodate generates reactive aldehyde groups that can be used for conjugation to amine-containing proteins. Reductive amination of oxidized HRP

Robert Hnasko (ed.), *ELISA: Methods and Protocols*, Methods in Molecular Biology, vol. 1318, DOI 10.1007/978-1-4939-2742-5_4, © Springer Science+Business Media New York 2015

Table 1
Chemical properties of heterobifunctional cross-linking reagents (sulfo-SMCC and SATA) used to conjugate and enzymatic reporter to an antibody

Chemical cross-linker	Sulfosuccinimidyl-4-(*N*-maleimidomethyl) cyclohexane-1-carboxylate, sodium salt	*N*-succinimidyl-S-acetyl-thioacetate
Synonym	Sulfo-SMCC	SATA
Empirical formula	$C_{16}H_{17}N_2NaO_5S$	$C_8H_9NO_5S$
Molecular weight	436.37	231.23
CAS number	92921-24-9	76931-93-6

to antibodies in the presence of sodium cyanoborohydride is one simple method to prepare highly active antibody-HRP conjugates [4].

Another well-established method is the use of heterobifunctional reagents (Table 1) such as the water-soluble (10 mg/mL) sulfosuccinimidyl-4-(N-maleimidomethyl)cyclohexane-1-carboxylate (sulfo-SMCC) and N-succinimidyl S-acetylthioacetate (SATA) to generate stable antibody-HRP conjugates as illustrated in Fig. 1. The sulfo-SMCC reagent contains an amine-reactive NHS ester on one end and a sulfhydryl-reactive maleimide group on the other end. In this type of reaction, the NHS ester of SMCC first creates sulfhydryl-reactive maleimide groups at the two HRP lysine residues, and cross-linking is achieved when mixed with sulfhydryl-containing antibody (SATA-modified) to create the final antibody-HRP conjugate [5–8]. Maleimides are maleic acid imides derived from the reaction of maleic anhydride and ammonia or amine derivatives. The double bond of the maleimides can undergo alkylation when reacted with sulfhydryl groups to form stable thioether bonds. Maleimide reactions are specific for thiols at pH 6.5–7.5 but may also undergo hydrolysis to an open maleamic acid that is unreactive to sulfhydryls, a process that occurs faster at a higher pH.

These heterobifunctional cross-linking reagents are used in controlled multistep protocols with great success to yield useful antibody-HRP conjugates. Sulfo-SMCC has a very stable maleimide functionality that affords the activation of either the HRP or antibody at amines reactive to the NHS ester end by limiting hydrolysis (*see* **Note 1**). This allows the resulting maleimide-activated intermediate to be purified from excess cross-linker, and other unwanted by-products, before mixing with the antibody and thereby exerting control over the extent of cross-linking while limiting unwanted polymerization of the conjugated protein.

The primary goal of antibody bioconjugation is the preparation of a stable antibody-enzyme conjugate that can serve as a target-directed reporter to detect or quantitate a specific antigen by immunoassay. The methods used to achieve this goal should yield an antibody that retains high antigen-binding affinity with robust enzymatic activity.

In this protocol, we describe the activation of HRP with sulfo-SMCC to create reactive maleimide groups for coupling to sulfhydryl groups introduced into antibodies by thiolation (*see* **Note 2**). The frequency of sulfhydryl occurrence in proteins is low when compared to amine or carboxylates, and this site limitation can restrict target antibody modification thereby increasing the probability that the antibody-HRP conjugate will retain antigen-binding activity.

SATA is a versatile thiolation reagent for introducing sulfhydryl groups into antibodies [6]. The active NHS ester end of SATA reacts with amino groups in proteins to form stable amide linkage resulting in a protein with an acetylated sulfhydryl that can be stored as stock solutions without degradation. Reactivity of the SATA-modified stock requires deacetylation prior to cross-linking by simple exposure to excess hydroxylamine. The SATA thiolation process results in nearly random attachment over the surface of the antibody structure, and it has been shown that as many as six SATA

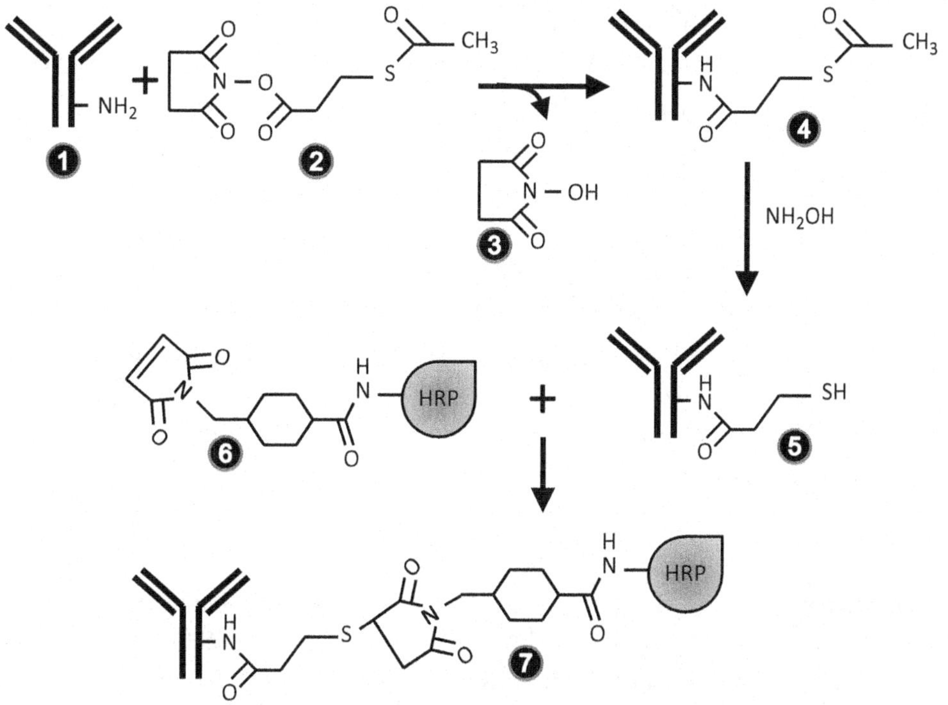

Fig. 1 Conjugation of SATA-modified antibody with sulfo-SMCC-activated HRP. Antibody amine groups ① modified with the NHS ester end of SATA ② generates an NHS ester ③ and antibody with amide bond derivatives with protected sulfhydryls ④. The acetylated thiols are unprotected with hydroxylamine at alkaline pH ⑤ and the reactive thiolated antibody combined with maleimide-activated HRP enzyme ⑥ that yields stable thioether cross-links and HRP-functionalized antibody ⑦

per antibody can have minimal effect in antigen-binding affinity. SATA creates sulfhydryl target groups necessary to conjugate with maleimide-activated HRP (*see* **Note 3**).

2 Materials

Microcentrifuge tubes.

Pipettes and tips.

pH meter.

Microcentrifuge.

Horseradish peroxidase.

0.1 M phosphate buffer (PB).

Sodium chloride (NaCl).

Ethylenediaminetetraacetic acid (EDTA).

Sulfo-SMCC reagent.

Gel filtration desalting columns packed with Sephadex G25.

Purified antibody for conjugation.

SATA reagent.

Dimethyl sulfoxide (DMSO) or dimethylformamide (DMF).

Hydroxylamine-HCL.

Protein-G agarose beads.

Protein-G binding buffer: sodium acetate (pH 5.0).

Protein-G elution buffer: 0.1 M glycine-HCL (pH 2–3).

Neutralization buffer: high-ionic strength alkaline buffer such as 1 M phosphate buffer (pH 7.5–9).

Dialysis bag/cassette or desalting column for buffer exchange.

Glycerol.

Thimerosal.

3 Methods

3.1 Activation of HRP with Sulfo-SMCC

1. Dissolve HRP in 0.1 M sodium phosphate with 150 mM NaCl at pH 7.2 (PBS) to a concentration of 20 mg/mL (*see* **Note 4**).

2. Add 3 mg of sulfo-SMCC to the HRP solution and vortex to mix, allow reaction to incubate at room temperature for 15 min, and then add another 3 mg of sulfo-SMCC and incubate an additional 15 min (*see* **Note 5**).

3. Immediately purify the maleimide-activated HRP away for excess cross-linker and reaction by-products by gel filtration

using a desalting column and PBS (Sephadex G25; 1/8th sample to bed volume) (*see* **Note 6**).

4. Collect 1 mL fractions and pool the first peak containing HRP (*see* **Note 7**).

5. Measure the protein concentration of the purified HRP and adjust to 10 mg/mL for the conjugation reaction. At this point, the maleimide-activated HRP should be used immediately for conjugation or freeze dry to preserve its maleimide activity.

3.2 Thiolation of Antibody

1. Freshly dissolve SATA in DMSO or DMF at 8 mg/mL.

2. Add 10–40 μL of SATA stock per 1 mg/mL of antibody in PB pH 6.5–7.5 (*see* **Note 8**).

3. React for 30 min at room temperature.

4. Purify SATA-modified antibody by gel filtration (Sephadex G25) using PBS pH 7.2 containing 1–10 mM EDTA (*see* **Note 9**).

3.3 Deacetylation of Sulfhydryl Groups on SATA-Modified Antibody

1. Freshly prepare 0.5 M hydroxylamine-HCL in PB (pH 7.2) with 10 mM EDTA.

2. Add 100 μL of hydroxylamine stock to each mL of SATA-modified antibody to achieve a final concentration of hydroxylamine in the antibody solution to 50 mM.

3. React for 2 h at room temperature.

4. Purify the deacetylated sulfhydryl-modified antibody by gel filtration (G25 Sephadex) using PBS with 1–10 mM EDTA pH 7.2 (*see* **Note 10**).

3.4 Bioconjugation of Sulfo-SMCC Maleimide-Activated HRP with SATA-Thiolated Antibody

1. Combine deacetylated sulfhydryl-modified antibody (SATA) with maleimide-activated HRP (sulfo-SMCC) using a ratio of 4:1 excess HRP enzyme to antibody (*see* **Note 11**).

2. Allow the reaction to proceed at room temperature for 2 h or overnight at 4 °C.

3.5 Immunoaffinity Purification of Antibody-HRP Conjugate by Liquid Chromatography

1. Prepare protein-G column by washing with 3–5× column volumes of protein-G binding buffer at a rate of 1 mL/min to remove preservative and exchange buffer and pH (*see* **Note 12**).

2. Dilute antibody-HRP conjugate with protein-G in binding buffer to adjust pH and pass over column 1–3× at a rate of 0.5–1 mL/min (*see* **Note 13**). Monitor protein absorbance at 280 nm using an in-line UV monitor as shown in Fig. 1 (*see* **Note 14**).

3. Pass at least 5× column volume of protein-G binding buffer at 1 mL/min to wash beads of residual unbound protein and return to baseline 280 nm absorbance values.

4. Apply protein-G elution buffer (0.1 M glycine-HCL, pH 2–3) at a rate of 1 mL/min and begin collecting 1 mL fractions into tube containing 0.1 mL of neutralization buffer (1 M PB buffer, pH 8.0). Monitor protein absorbance at 280 nm UV to identify desorption of the IgG from the resin as an A_{280} protein peak and collect fractions until baseline protein measurement is achieved (*see* **Note 15**).

5. Determine protein concentration of each elution fraction by measuring absorbance at 280 nm or performing a protein assay such as Bradford or BCA.

6. Evaluate affinity-purified elution fractions for antibody and HRP activity by ELISA.

7. Pool peak fractions and dialyze against desired buffer. Centrifugal concentrators can be used to increase desired concentration of purified antibody-HRP. The addition of 10 % glycerol to the final antibody-HRP stock is useful for long-term storage (*see* **Note 16**).

4   Notes

1. The enhanced stability of sulfo-SMCC maleimide group and water solubility is mediated by negatively charged sulfonate on its sulfo-NHS ring. Ready to use SMCC-activated HRP can be commercially purchased from multiple vendors.

2. An alternate way to create an available sulfhydryl group is by disruption of the disulfide bridge at the hinge region of the IgG with reducing reagents such as dithiothreitol (DTT), 2-ME (2-mercaptoethanol), or Tris (2-carboxyethyl) phosphine hydrochloride (TCEP) resulting in two heavy-light chain antibody halves. This process can result in a diminished affinity and should be evaluated carefully to determine suitability for downstream applications.

3. The introduction of sulfhydryl groups avoids the need for reducing reagents to alter native sites within the antibody structure that can adversely affect antigen affinity.

4. The more highly concentrated the HRP enzyme, the more efficient the modification of the reaction.

5. A 40–80 M excess of cross-linker to protein should be used.

6. Avoid dialysis of the reaction as the maleimide activity will be lost during the process.

7. On a column, HRP can be visually observed as it flows through the column by the dark color of its heme ring.

8. Use a ~10–50-fold molar excess of SATA to antibody. A 12-fold molar excess is a useful starting concentration of SATA.

Increasing SATA concentration results in more potential HRP conjugation reactions per molecule of antibody. Do not exceed 10 % DMSO in the aqueous reaction mixture.

9. At this stage, the SATA-modified antibody with stable acetylated sulfhydryl groups can be stored as stock solutions until needed.

10. Deacetylated sulfhydryl-modified antibody should be used immediately for conjugation to HRP to prevent loss of sulfhydryl content via disulfide bond formation.

11. This ratio of HRP to antibody may need to be adjusted to maximize conjugation.

12. Purification of antibody-HRP conjugate from unconjugated excess HRP by immunoaffinity chromatography is useful to decrease immunoassay signal background.

13. Passing fluid over column can be accomplished by either gravity flow, manually pushing fluid by way of Luer-lock syringe, or peristaltic pump. The antibody binding capacity of protein-G is approximately 6–8 mg of mouse IgG per mL of resin.

14. In-line monitoring of 280 nm absorbance is a convenient way of monitoring protein concentration in real time. This provides a rapid assessment of column performance and antibody elution without the need for downstream evaluation of individual fractions. If this is not available, measuring the protein concentration of each individual labeled fraction can provide the evaluation at the end of the run. Estimate of IgG concentration based on 280 nm absorbance; $1.43\ A_{280} = 1$ mg/mL.

15. An alternative to collecting individual elution fractions is by using a single tube too harvest the entire IgG peak. This can be accomplished by monitoring the A_{280} and collecting just the volume associated with the IgG protein peak. This can maximize antibody concentration by reducing total volume.

16. One can include an antibacterial agent such as 0.05 % thimerosal in the final antibody solution, but avoid sodium azide as it can inhibit HRP.

References

1. Brinkley M (1992) A brief survey of methods for preparing protein conjugates with dyes, haptens, and cross-linking reagents. Bioconjug Chem 3:2–13

2. Veitch NC (2004) Horseradish peroxidase: a modern view of a classic enzyme. Phytochemistry 65:249–259

3. Marquette CA, Blum LJ (2009) Chemiluminescent enzyme immunoassays: a review of bioanalytical applications. Bioanalysis 7:1259–1269

4. Wolfe CA, Hage DS (1995) Studies on the rate and control of antibody oxidation by periodate. Anal Biochem 23:123–130

5. Bieniarz C, Husain M, Barnes G et al (1996) Extended length heterobifunctional coupling agents for protein conjugations. Bioconjug Chem 7:88–95

6. Duncan RJ, Weston PD, Wrigglesworth R (1983) A new reagent which may be used to introduce sulfhydryl groups into proteins, and its use in the preparation of conjugates for immunoassay. Anal Biochem 132:68–73

7. Hashida S, Imagawa M, Inoue S et al (1984) More useful maleimide compounds for the conjugation of Fab' to horseradish peroxidase through thiol groups in the hinge. J Appl Biochem 6:56–63

8. Peeters JM, Hazendonk TG, Beuvery EC et al (1989) Comparison of four bifunctional reagents for coupling peptides to proteins and the effect of the three moieties on the immunogenicity of the conjugates. J Immunol Methods 120:133–143

Chapter 5

Indirect ELISA

Alice V. Lin

Abstract

The enzyme-linked immunosorbent assay (ELISA) is a simple and rapid technique for detecting and quantitating antibodies or antigens attached to a solid surface. Being one of the most sensitive immunoassays, ELISA offers commercial value in laboratory research, diagnostic of disease biomarkers, and quality control in various industries. This technique utilizes an enzyme-linked antibody binding to a surface-attached antigen. Subsequently, a substrate is added to produce either a color change or light signal correlating to the amount of the antigen present in the original sample. This chapter provides the procedures required for carrying out indirect ELISA, one of the many forms of ELISA, to detect polystyrene-immobilized antigen. Methodological approaches to optimize this assay technique are also described, a prerequisite for automation and multiplexing.

Key words ELISA, Immunoassay, Antibody, Chemiluminescence, Chessboard titration

1 Introduction

First described by Engvall and Perlmann, the enzyme-linked immunosorbent assay (ELISA) is a technique based on an enzyme-labeled antibody capable of detecting and quantifying protein immobilized to a solid surface [1]. ELISA is traditionally performed in 96-well or 384-well polystyrene plates where antigen or antibody binds through passive absorption [2]. As the technology advances, variations to ELISA such as ELISPOT and in-cell ELISA emerge. Multiplex microarray ELISA significantly improves the traditional technique by allowing each well to screen multiple analytes with a limit of detection 1,000-fold higher than traditional ELISA [3]. The term ELISA now loosely applies to assays involving antibody detection of analyte.

Traditional ELISA can be performed in four different formats, direct, indirect, sandwich, and competitive. In indirect ELISA, the antigen of interest is immobilized to a 96-well or 384-well polystyrene microtiter plates by passive absorption [2]. A blocking buffer is added to saturate all unbound sites in the well followed by

Robert Hnasko (ed.), *ELISA: Methods and Protocols*, Methods in Molecular Biology, vol. 1318,
DOI 10.1007/978-1-4939-2742-5_5, © Springer Science+Business Media New York 2015

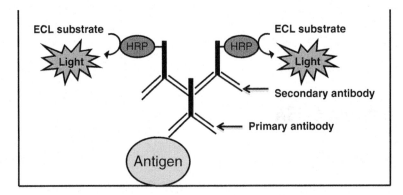

Fig. 1 Schematic diagram to illustrate the principle of indirect ELISA in generating light signal from plate-immobilized antigen

incubation with an unlabeled primary antibody specific for the antigen. An anti-species enzyme-conjugated secondary antibody is subsequently added to bind to the primary antibody. Typically, the secondary antibody is conjugated to horseradish peroxidase (HRP) and detected with enhanced chemiluminescent substrate (ECL) [4, 5]. Another common method is to utilize biotin-coupled primary antibody and enzyme-conjugated streptavidin secondary antibody. In both cases, the substrate produces measurable unit corresponding directly to the amount of antigen present in the well.

This chapter describes the methodology of performing indirect ELISA on 96-well polystyrene plates using HRP-conjugated secondary antibody followed by detection with enhanced chemiluminescent substrate (ECL) depicted in Fig. 1. In addition, procedures to optimize the antigen, primary antibody, and secondary antibody by chessboard titration are also provided. Similar to direct ELISA, indirect ELISA is useful for antibody screening, epitope mapping, and protein quantification [6, 7]. The secondary antibody serves to enhance the signal of the primary antibody thus making it more sensitive than direct ELISA. However, it also produces a higher background signal and potentially decreases the overall net signal. As with any immunoassay, optimization is required.

2   Materials

1. Buffers.

    (a) Binding solution: 0.2 M carbonate-bicarbonate, pH 9.4 (Thermo Scientific, Rockford, IL, USA).

    (b) Blocking solution: 10 % nonfat dry milk in TBST.

    (c) Wash solution: Tris-buffered saline (pH 7.4) with 0.1 % (v/v) Tween 20 (TBST).

    (d) Dilution buffer: 1 % nonfat dry milk in TBST.

2. Antigen and antibodies.

   (a) Antigen of interest partially purified or purified.

   (b) Primary antibody to the antigen of interest.

   (c) Secondary antibody conjugated to HRP (usually anti-species polyclonal).

   (d) Substrate: enhanced chemiluminescent (ECL) HRP substrate (Thermo Scientific, Rockford, IL, USA) (*see* **Note 1**).

3. Supplies and instruments.

   (a) White 96-well plates (Greiner 655074 or Nunc Maxisorp® 436110) (*see* **Note 2**).

   (b) 96-well plate cover or adhesive seal.

   (c) 96-well plate reader: PerkinElmer VICTOR™ X3 Multilabel Plate Reader (PerkinElmer, Waltham, MA).

   (d) ELISA plate washer (optional).

   (e) Titer plate shaker.

3 Methods

3.1 Antigen Immobilization

1. Dilute antigen in binding solution. Antigen should be diluted into a final concentration ranging from 1–100 μg/ml [8] (*see* Subheading 3.5 for optimization).

2. Add 100 μl of diluted antigen into each well. Seal the plate with cover or adhesive and incubate for 2 h at room temperature or overnight at 4 °C (*see* **Note 3**).

3. Aspirate off the antigen and wash four times with 200 μl wash solution either by hand or ELISA plate washer. This step washes off any unbound antigen.

4. Optional step: short chemical denaturation (*see* **Note 4**) [9].

   (a) Prepare 1 M solution of guanidine-HCl.

   (b) Add 100 μl to each well and incubate for 1 h.

   (c) Aspirate off the antigen and wash four times with 200 μl of wash solution either by hand or ELISA plate washer.

3.2 Blocking

1. Add 200 μl of blocking solution into each well and incubate at room temperature for 30 min to overnight (*see* **Note 5**).

2. Aspirate off the blocking solution. It is not necessary to wash the plate at this point.

3.3 Incubation with Primary Antibody

1. Dilute primary antibody in dilution buffer. Primary antibody should be diluted into a final concentration of 1 μg/ml or follow manufacturer's instruction.

2. Add 100 μl of diluted HRP-conjugated antibody into each well. Seal the plate with cover or adhesive and incubate at room temperature for 1 h.

3. Aspirate off the antibody and wash four times with 200 μl wash solution either by hand or ELISA plate washer.

3.4 Immobilized Antigen Detection by HRP-Conjugated Secondary Antibody

1. Dilute HRP-conjugated secondary antibody in dilution buffer. HRP-conjugated antibody can be commercially purchased and is usually anti-species to the primary antibody. The secondary antibody should be diluted into a final concentration following manufacturer's instruction or 1:10 K of 1 mg/ml stock.

2. Add 100 μl of diluted HRP-conjugated antibody into each well. Seal the plate with cover or adhesive and incubate at room temperature for 1 h.

3. Aspirate off the antibody and wash four times with 200 μl wash solution either by hand or ELISA plate washer.

4. Prepare ECL substrate according to manufacturer's instruction.

5. Add 50–100 μl of substrate into each well.

6. Place the ELISA plate on a titer plate shaker and incubate for 2 min at room temperature.

7. Read the light signal (relative light units) using PerkinElmer VICTOR™ X3 Multilabel Plate Reader.

3.5 Optimization by Chessboard Titration

It is essential to optimize each component of indirect ELISA to avoid prozone or hook effect and generate reliable data [10] . Chessboard titration is a common method allowing the titration of two reagents at a time as shown in Fig. 2. This section describes the steps for optimization of antigen, primary antibody, and HRP-conjugated secondary antibody concentrations.

3.6 Chessboard Titration of Antigen and Primary Antibody

3.6.1 Titration of Antigen

1. Fill columns 2–12 with 100 μl of binding solution.

2. Dilute antigen in binding solution into a final concentration of 100 μg/ml for partially purified protein sample or 10 μg/ml for purified small peptides.

3. Add 200 μl of diluted antigen sample into all eight wells of column 1.

4. Aspirate off 100 μl of diluted antigen from wells in column 1 and transfer to wells in column 2. Gently pipette up and down three times to mix the content of the well.

5. Repeat **step 4** and perform dilute antigen from columns 2–11. Leave column 12 with binding buffer only.

6. Seal the plate with cover or adhesive and incubate for 2 h at room temperature or overnight at 4 °C.

7. Aspirate off the antigen and wash four times with 200 μl wash solution either by hand or ELISA plate washer.

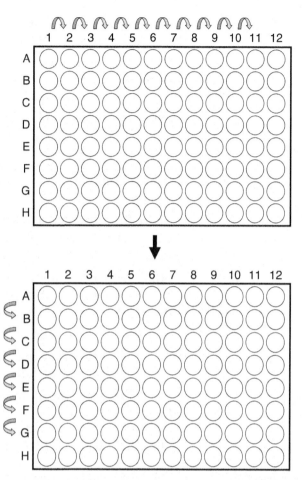

Fig. 2 Suggested layout of chessboard titration optimizing the concentrations of antigen, primary antibody, and secondary antibody in 96-well plates. The antigen is titrated across from *columns 1–11* followed by the titration of primary antibody from *rows A–G*. Once the optimal concentration of the antigen is determined, a second chessboard titration should be performed titrating the primary antibody from *columns 1–11* and the secondary antibody from *rows A–G*

8. Add 200 μl of blocking solution into each well and incubate at room temperature for 30 min to overnight.

9. Aspirate off the blocking solution. It is not necessary to wash the plate at this point.

3.6.2 Titration of the Primary Antibody

1. Fill rows B–H with 100 μl of dilution buffer.

2. Dilute the primary antibody in dilution buffer into a final concentration of 1 μg/ml.

3. Add 200 μl of diluted antibody into all 12 wells of row A.

4. Aspirate off 100 μl of diluted antibody from row A and transfer to row B. Gently pipette up and down three times to mix the content of the well.

5. Repeat **step 4** and titrate primary antibody from row B to row G. Leave row H with dilution buffer only.

6. Seal the plate with cover or adhesive and incubate for 1 h at room temperature.

7. Aspirate off the antigen and wash four times with 200 μl wash solution either by hand or ELISA plate washer.

3.6.3 Detection with HRP-Conjugated Secondary Antibody

1. Dilute HRP-conjugated secondary antibody in dilution buffer. The secondary antibody should be diluted into a final concentration following manufacturer's instruction or 1:10 K of 1 mg/ml stock.

2. Add 100 μl of diluted HRP-conjugated antibody into each well. Seal the plate with cover or adhesive and incubate at room temperature for 1 h.

3. Aspirate off the antibody and wash four times with 200 μl wash solution either by hand or ELISA plate washer.

4. Prepare ECL substrate according to manufacturer's instruction.

5. Add 50–100 μl of substrate into each well.

6. Place the ELISA plate on a titer plate shaker and incubate for 2 min at room temperature.

7. Read the light signal (relative light units, RLU) using PerkinElmer VICTOR™ X3 Multilabel Plate Reader. An example of RLU values in a chessboard titration is shown in Fig. 3 for sample outcome and interpretation.

3.7 Chessboard Titration of Primary Antibody and HRP-Conjugated Secondary Antibody

3.7.1 Titration of Primary Antibody

1. Dilute antigen in binding solution. Antigen should be diluted into the optimal concentration obtained from chessboard titration of antigen and primary antibody. 12.5 μg/ml for partially purified protein sample and 1.25 μg/ml for purified peptides from Fig. 3.

5. Add 100 μl of diluted antigen into all 96 wells. Seal the plate with cover or adhesive and incubate for 2 h at room temperature or overnight at 4 °C.

6. Aspirate off the antigen and wash four times with 200 μl wash solution either by hand or ELISA plate washer. This step washes off any unbound antigen.

7. Add 200 μl of blocking solution into each well and incubate at room temperature for 30 min to overnight.

3. Aspirate off the blocking solution. It is not necessary to wash the plate at this point.

4. Fill columns 2–11 with 100 μl of dilution buffer.

5. Dilute primary antibody in dilution buffer into a final concentration of 1 μg/ml.

6. Add 200 μl of diluted primary antibody into all eight wells of column 1.

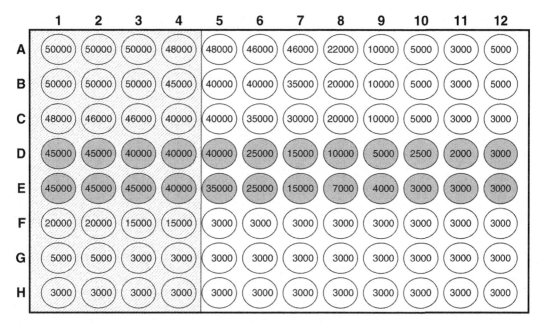

Fig. 3 This illustrates a sample outcome of chessboard titration. *Columns 1–4* are *boxed* indicating the titration of antigen does not significantly affect the output signal. The optimal antigen concentration is 12.5 µg/ml for partially purified protein sample and 1.25 µg/ml for purified peptides. This is the minimal amount of antigen required to generate the maximum signal in this assay. The primary antibody gives the greatest range of titration when used at 0.06–0.125 µg/ml as shown in *rows D* and *E*. This is the optimal primary antibody concentration in this assay

7. Aspirate off 100 µl of diluted primary antibody from wells in column 1 and transfer to wells in column 2. Gently pipette up and down three times to mix the content of the well.

8. Repeat **step 7** and dilute primary antibody from columns 2–11. Leave column 12 with dilution buffer only.

9. Seal the plate with cover or adhesive and incubate for 1 h at room temperature.

10. Aspirate off the antigen and wash four times with 200 µl wash solution either by hand or ELISA plate washer. This step washes off any unbound primary antibody.

3.7.2 Titration of HRP-Conjugated Secondary Antibody

1. Fill rows B–H with 100 µl of dilution buffer.

2. Dilute the HRP-conjugated antibody in dilution buffer into a final concentration fourfold higher than recommended by the manufacturer or 1:2,500 of 1 mg/ml stock solution.

3. Add 200 µl of diluted antibody into all 12 wells of row A.

4. Aspirate off 100 µl of diluted secondary antibody from row A and transfer to row B. Gently pipette up and down three times to mix the content of the well.

5. Repeat **step 4** and titrate secondary antibody from row B to row G. Leave row H with dilution buffer only.

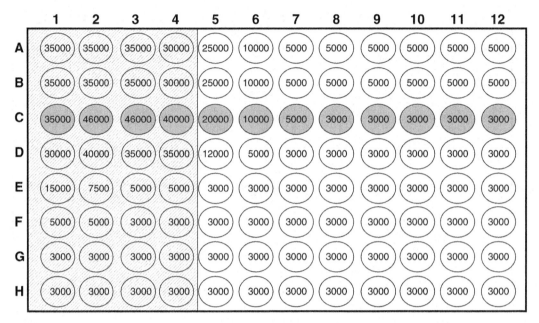

Fig. 4 Based on the result from Fig. 3, 12.5 µg/ml of partially purified protein sample or 1.25 µg/ml of purified peptides is used to coat the plate. Primary antibody is titrated from *rows 1–11*, and no significant difference in relative light unit is observed from *rows 1–4*. This indicates the primary antibody can be diluted down to 0.125 µg/ml without much loss in signal, consistent with the result from Fig. 3. *Row C* is highlighted to indicate the optimal concentration of the secondary antibody, the minimal amount required without loss in signal. This reflects 1× of manufacturer's suggested dilution or 1:10 K of 1 mg/ml stock solution

6. Seal the plate with cover or adhesive and incubate for 1 h at room temperature.

7. Aspirate off the antigen and wash four times with 200 µl wash solution either by hand or ELISA plate washer.

8. Prepare ECL substrate according to manufacturer's instruction.

9. Add 50–100 µl of substrate into each well.

10. Place the ELISA plate on a titer plate shaker and incubate for 2 min at room temperature.

11. Read the light signal (relative light units) using PerkinElmer VICTOR™ X3 Multilabel Plate Reader. An example of RLU values in a chessboard titration is shown in Fig. 4 for sample outcome and interpretation.

4   Notes

1. Sodium azide and compounds containing cyanides and sulfides are inhibitors of HRP. Therefore, reagents used in ELISA should be free of these compounds. 0.01 % thimerosal can be used as an alternative antibacterial reagent.

2. Chemiluminescent HRP-based assays require black or white opaque plates to minimize leaching of light into neighboring wells. White plates are preferred to amplify signal. ELISA plates are usually flat bottomed and made from polystyrene or polyvinyl chloride. Plates are manufactured to minimize edge effect, but each batch should still be tested to ensure consistency.

3. Most protein antigens in binding solution can be refrigerated in plate wells for up to a week without much loss in signal. Care should be taken to seal individual wells to prevent evaporation. This may be convenient for screening large quantities of wells. However, the stability of individual antigen on ELISA plates should be tested before proceeding with long-term refrigeration.

4. Adding guanidine-HCl allows partial unfolding of antigen passively absorbed to plate to creating more antibody-binding epitopes. This step is generally not required since most ELISA assays give robust signal. In addition, some antibodies may be sensitive to guanidine-HCl. If this is the case, 1 M urea or 1 M SDS can be used as alternatives.

5. 10 % nonfat dry milk in TBST is a typical blocking reagent used in ELISA. However, it can nonspecifically react with some antibodies. Alternative blocking agents include BSA, fish gelatin in PBS, or commercial nonprotein-based blocks. A nonprotein-based block has the advantage of not containing IgG which potentially make nonspecific interaction with antibodies.

References

1. Engvall E, Perlmann P (1971) Enzyme-linked immunosorbent assay (ELISA). Quantitative assay of immunoglobulin G. Immunochemistry 8:871–874

2. Stevens PW, Hansberry MR, Kelso DM (1995) Assessment of adsorption and adhesion of proteins to polystyrene microwells by sequential enzyme-linked immunosorbent assay analysis. Anal Biochem 225:197–205

3. Desmet C, Blum LJ, Marquette CA (2013) Multiplex microarray ELISA versus classical ELISA, a comparison study of pollutant sensing for environmental analysis. Environ Sci Process Impacts 10:1876–1882

4. Fan A, Cao Z, Li H et al (2009) Chemiluminescence platforms in immunoassay and DNA analyses. Anal Sci 25:5875–5897

5. Gan SD, Patel KR (2013) Enzyme immunoassay and enzyme-linked immunosorbent assay. J Invest Dermatol 133:e12

6. Hornbeck P (2001) Enzyme-linked immunosorbent assays. Curr Protoc Immunol Chapter 2: Unit 2.1. doi: 10.1002/0471142735. im0201s01

7. Natarajan S, Remick DG (2008) The ELISA standard save: calculation of sample concentrations in assays with a failed standard curve. J Immunol Methods 336:242–245

8. Underwood PA, Steele JG (1991) Practical limitations of estimation of protein adsorption to polymer surfaces. J Immunol Methods 142:83–94

9. Hnasko R, Lin A, McGarvey JA et al (2011) A rapid method to improve protein detection by indirect ELISA. Biochem Biophys Res Commun 410:726–731

10. Vos Q, Klasen EA, Haaijman JJ (1987) The effect of divalent and univalent binding on antibody titration curves in solid-phase ELISA. J Immunol Methods 103:47–54

Chapter 6

Direct ELISA

Alice V. Lin

Abstract

First described by Engvall and Perlmann, the enzyme-linked immunosorbent assay (ELISA) is a rapid and sensitive method for detection and quantitation of an antigen using an enzyme-labeled antibody. Besides routine laboratory usage, ELISA has been utilized in medical field and food industry as diagnostic and quality control tools. Traditionally performed in 96-well or 384-well polystyrene plates, the technology has expanded to other platforms with increase in automation. Depending on the antigen epitope and availability of specific antibody, there are variations in ELISA setup. The four basic formats are direct, indirect, sandwich, and competitive ELISAs. Direct ELISA is the simplest format requiring an antigen and an enzyme-conjugated antibody specific to the antigen. This chapter describes the individual steps for detection of a plate-bound antigen using a horseradish peroxidase (HRP)-conjugated antibody and luminol-based enhanced chemiluminescence (ECL) substrate. The methodological approach to optimize the assay by chessboard titration is also provided.

Key words ELISA, Immunoassay, Antibody, Chemiluminescence, Chessboard titration

1 Introduction

The enzyme-linked immunosorbent assay (ELISA) is a technique based on an enzyme-labeled antibody capable of detecting an antigen immobilized to a solid surface, most commonly 96-well or 384-well polystyrene plates [1]. This high-throughput assay relies on unbound materials to be washed off between steps, allowing detection of the enzyme-labeled antibody attached to the antigen. The most commonly used enzymes are alkaline phosphatase (AP) and horseradish peroxidase (HRP). HRP is generally preferred for its lower detection limit [2]. As the technique advances, ELISA has been adopted to other platforms for multiplexing, and the term ELISA has evolved to loosely refer to assays involving antibody detection of analyte [3].

As with any immunoassay, the key to ELISA is the antibody. Antibody affinity and avidity determine the sensitivity and specificity of the assay. Antibody can be employed in several ways in an ELISA assay. It can be directly conjugated to an enzyme to detect

Robert Hnasko (ed.), *ELISA: Methods and Protocols*, Methods in Molecular Biology, vol. 1318,
DOI 10.1007/978-1-4939-2742-5_6, © Springer Science+Business Media New York 2015

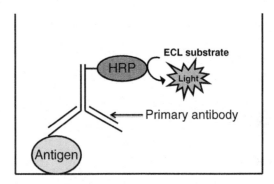

Fig. 1 Schematic diagram to illustrate the principle of direct ELISA in generating light signal from plate-immobilized antigen

plate-immobilized antigen, a form known as direct ELISA. Alternately, a secondary antibody can be used to amplify the signal of the primary antibody bound to the antigen, also known as indirect ELISA. A third method immobilizes antibody onto a plate to capture an antigen in solution followed by detecting with another enzyme-conjugated antibody recognizing a different epitope of the same antigen. This popular method, also known as sandwich ELISA, gives the greatest sensitivity for detecting a specific antigen in a complex sample. A fourth format, also known as competitive ELISA, utilizes a mixture of antibody-antigen and free antibody in liquid phase to interact with plate-immobilized antigens [4].

This chapter provides the methodology for performing direct ELISA as illustrated in Fig. 1 and optimizing performance by chessboard titration. In the direct ELISA, the antigen of interest in fluid phase is immobilized to a microtiter plate through passive absorption [5]. A blocking buffer is added to saturate all unbound sites followed by the binding of enzyme-labeled antibody. Antibody in direct ELISA can be monoclonal or polyclonal. A substrate is added to generate a color change or emit light indicating the presence of antigen. Direct ELISA is useful for qualitative or quantitative antigen detection in a sample, antibody screening, and epitope mapping [6]. Since only one antibody is involved, there is no cross-reactivity with secondary antibody, and the assay can be performed in less amount of time compared to other ELISA methods.

2 Materials

1. Buffers.
    (a) Binding solution: 0.2 M carbonate-bicarbonate, pH 9.4.
    (b) Wash solution: Tris-buffered saline (pH 7.4) with 0.1 % (v/v) Tween 20 (TBST).

(c) Blocking solution: 10 % nonfat dry milk in TBST.

(d) Dilution buffer: 1 % nonfat dry milk in TBST.

2. Antigen and antibodies.

(a) Antigen of interest partially purified or purified.

(b) Primary antibody, monoclonal or polyclonal, conjugated to horseradish peroxidase (HRP). Antibody can be purchased in the HRP-conjugated form or self-conjugate with Lightning-Link™ HRP Conjugation Kit (Innova Biosciences, Cambridge, UK) (*see* **Note 1**).

(c) Substrate: enhanced chemiluminescent (ECL) HRP substrate (*see* **Note 2**).

3. Supplies and instruments.

(a) White 96-well plates (Greiner 655074 or Nunc Maxisorp® 436110) (*see* **Note 3**).

(b) 96-well plate cover or adhesive seal.

(c) 96-well plate reader: PerkinElmer VICTOR™ X3 Multilabel Plate Reader (PerkinElmer, Waltham, MA).

(d) ELISA plate washer (optional).

(e) Titer plate shaker.

3 Methods

3.1 Antigen Immobilization

1. Dilute antigen in binding buffer. Antigen should be diluted into a final concentration ranging from 1–100 µg/ml [7] (*see* Subheading 3.4 for optimization).

2. Add 100 µl of diluted antigen into each well. Seal the plate with cover or adhesive and incubate for 2 h at room temperature or overnight at 4 °C (*see* **Note 4**).

3. Aspirate off the antigen and wash four times with 200 µl wash solution either by hand or ELISA plate washer. This step washes off any unbound antigen.

4. Optional step: short chemical denaturation (*see* **Note 5**) [8].

(a) Prepare 1 M solution of guanidine-HCl.

(b) Add 100 µl to each well and incubate for 1 h.

(c) Aspirate off the denaturant and wash four times with 200 µl of wash solution either by hand or ELISA plate washer.

3.2 Blocking

1. Add 200 µl of blocking solution into each well and incubate at room temperature for 30 min to overnight (*see* **Note 6**).

2. Aspirate off the blocking solution. It is not necessary to wash the plate at this point.

3.3 Immobilized Antigen Detection by Labeled Antibody

1. Dilute HRP-conjugated antibody in dilution buffer. HRP-conjugated antibody should be diluted into a final concentration of 1 µg/ml or follow manufacturer's instruction.

2. Add 100 µl of diluted HRP-conjugated antibody into each well. Seal the plate with cover or adhesive and incubate at room temperature for 1 h.

3. Aspirate off the antibody and wash four times with 200 µl wash solution either by hand or ELISA plate washer.

4. Prepare ECL substrate according to manufacturer's instruction.

5. Add 50–100 µl of substrate into each well.

6. Place the plate on a titer plate shaker and incubate for 2 min at room temperature.

7. Read the light signal using PerkinElmer VICTOR™ X3 Multilabel Plate Reader.

3.4 Optimization by Chessboard Titration

A common phenomenon observed in ELISA is the prozone or hook effect [9]. This occurs when either the antigen or the antibody is used at high concentration but gives false low signal. A simple method of optimizing antigen and antibody concentrations is by chessboard titration illustrated in Fig. 2.

Titration of Antigen

1. Fill columns 2–11 with 100 µl of binding solution.

2. Dilute antigen in binding solution into a final concentration of 100 µg/ml for partially purified sample or 10 µg/ml for purified peptides.

3. Add 200 µl of diluted antigen into A1–H1.

4. Aspirate off 100 µl of diluted antigen from wells in column 1 and transfer to wells in column 2. Gently pipette up and down three times to mix the content of the well.

5. Repeat **step 4** and dilute antigen from columns 2–11. Leave column 12 with binding buffer only.

6. Seal the plate with cover or adhesive and incubate for 2 h at room temperature or overnight at 4 °C.

7. Aspirate off the antigen and wash four times with 200 µl wash solution either by hand or ELISA plate washer. This step washes off any unbound antigen.

8. Add 200 µl of blocking solution into each well and incubate at room temperature for 30 min to overnight.

9. Aspirate off the blocking solution. It is not necessary to wash the plate at this point.

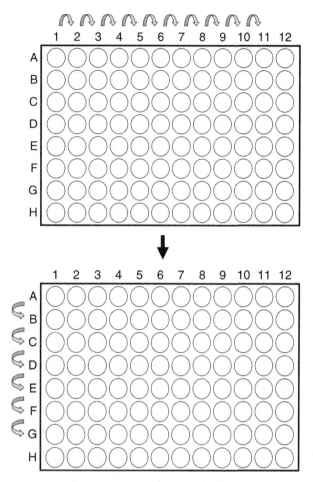

Fig. 2 Suggested layout of chessboard titration optimizing the concentrations of antigen and antibody in 96-well plates. Antigen is titrated across from *columns 1–11* followed by antibody being titrated down from *rows A* through *G*

Titration of Antibody

1. Fill rows B–H with 100 μl of dilution buffer.

2. Dilute HRP-conjugated antibody in dilution buffer into a final concentration of 1 μg/ml.

3. Add 200 μl of diluted antibody into all 12 wells of row A.

4. Aspirate off 100 μl of diluted antibody from row A and transfer to row B. Gently pipette up and down three times to mix the content of the well.

5. Repeat **step 4** and dilute antibody from row B to row G. Leave row H with dilution buffer only.

6. Seal the plate with cover or adhesive and incubate for 1 h at room temperature.

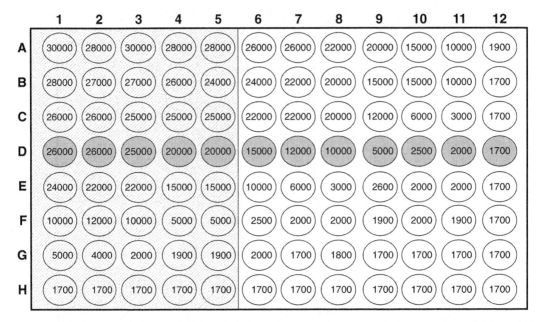

Fig. 3 Sample outcome of chessboard titration with results shown in relative light units (RLU). *Columns 1–5* are *boxed* showing no significant change in RLU indicating the optimal concentration for antigen is 6.25 µg/ml for partially purified protein sample and 0.625 µg/ml for purified peptide. This is the lowest amount of antigen required to produce the maximum amount of signal in this ELISA setup. *Row D* is highlighted to indicate the antibody concentration that gives the greatest range of titration. *Row D* corresponds to 0.125 µg/ml of antibody and titrates from *D5–D11*

7. Aspirate off the antigen and wash four times with 200 µl wash solution either by hand or ELISA plate washer. This step washes off any unbound antibody.

8. Add 50–100 µl of substrate into each well.

9. Place the ELISA plate on a titer plate shaker and incubate for 2 min at room temperature.

10. Read the light signal using PerkinElmer VICTOR™ X3 Multilabel Plate Reader.

11. *See* Fig. 3 for interpretation of chessboard titration data.

4   Notes

1. HRP-conjugated antibodies should be stored at –20 °C in 50 % glycerol to prevent decrease in signal.

2. Sodium azide and compounds containing cyanides and sulfides are inhibitors of HRP. Therefore, reagents used in ELISA should be free of these compounds. 0.01 % thimerosal can be used as an alternative antibacterial reagent.

3. Chemiluminescent HRP-based assays require black or white opaque plates to minimize leaching of light into neighboring wells. White plates are preferred to amplify light signal. ELISA plates are usually flat bottomed and made from polystyrene or polyvinyl chloride. Plates are manufactured to minimize edge effect, but each batch should still be tested to ensure consistency.

4. Most protein antigens in binding solution can be refrigerated in plate wells for up to a week without much loss in signal. Care should be taken to seal individual wells to prevent evaporation. This may be convenient for screening large quantities of wells. However, the stability of individual antigen on ELISA plates should be tested before proceeding with long-term refrigeration.

5. Proteins passively absorbed to polystyrene plates result in random orientation, and aggregation may occur affecting the presentation of epitopes to antibody. Adding guanidine-HCl allows partial unfolding of antigen to unmask epitopes covered by aggregation. However, this step also destroys conformational epitopes. In addition, some antibodies may be sensitive to guanidine-HCl. If this is the case, 1 M urea or 1 M SDS can be used as alternatives.

6. 10 % nonfat dry milk in TBST is a typical blocking reagent used in ELISA. However, it can nonspecifically react with some antibodies. Alternative blocking agents such as BSA, fish gelatin, or commercial nonprotein-based blocks can be used. A nonprotein-based block has the advantage of not containing IgG which potentially makes nonspecific interaction with antibodies.

References

1. Engvall E, Perlmann P (1971) Enzyme-linked immunosorbent assay (ELISA). Quantitative assay of immunoglobulin G. Immunochemistry 8:871–874

2. Fan A, Cao Z, Li H et al (2009) Chemiluminescence platforms in immunoassay and DNA analyses. Anal Sci 25:5875–5897

3. Czerkinsky CC, Nilsson LA, Nygren H et al (1983) A solid-phase enzyme-linked immunospot (ELISPOT) assay for enumeration of specific antibody-secreting cells. J Immunol Methods 65:109–121

4. Crowther JR (1995) ELISA. Theory and practice. Methods Mol Biol 42:1–218

5. Stevens PW, Hansberry MR, Kelso DM (1995) Assessment of adsorption and adhesion of proteins to polystyrene microwells by sequential enzyme-linked immunosorbent assay analysis. Anal Biochem 225:197–205

6. Hornbeck P (2001) Enzyme-linked immunosorbent assays. Curr Protoc Immunol Chapter 2: Unit 2.1. doi:10.1002/0471142735.im0201s01

7. Underwood PA, Steele JG (1991) Practical limitations of estimation of protein adsorption to polymer surfaces. J Immunol Methods 142:83–94

8. Hnasko R, Lin A, McGarvey JA et al (2011) A rapid method to improve protein detection by indirect ELISA. Biochem Biophys Res Commun 410:726–731

9. Vos Q, Klasen EA, Haaijman JJ (1987) The effect of divalent and univalent binding on antibody titration curves in solid-phase ELISA. J Immunol Methods 103:47–54

A Double-Sandwich ELISA for Identification of Monoclonal Antibodies Suitable for Sandwich Immunoassays

Larry H. Stanker and Robert M. Hnasko

Abstract

The sandwich immunoassay (sELISA) is an invaluable technique for concentrating, detecting, and quantifying target antigens. The two critical components required are a capture antibody and a detection antibody, each binding a different epitope on the target antigen. The specific antibodies incorporated into the test define most of the performance parameters of any subsequent immunoassay regardless of the assay format: traditional ELISA, lateral-flow immunoassay, various bead-based assays, antibody-based biosensors, or the reporting label. Here we describe an approach for identifying monoclonal antibodies (mAbs) suitable for use as capture antibodies and detector antibodies in a sELISA targeting bacterial protein toxins. The approach was designed for early identification of monoclonal antibodies (mAbs), in the initial hybridoma screen.

Key words Capture immunoassay, Hybridoma, Monoclonal antibody, sELISA, Lateral-flow immunoassay, Bacterial toxins, Botulinum neurotoxin

1 Introduction

The enzyme-linked immunosorbent assay (ELISA) [1] has enjoyed application in many areas because of its high specificity and sensitivity. Many variations are known including the indirect ELISA, competitive ELISA, the antibody-sandwich ELISA, antibody-capture ELISA, and the double antibody-sandwich ELISA. One of the most useful immunoassay formats is the sandwich ELISA designed for detection of soluble antigens. The difference between a capture ELISA and a sandwich ELISA is that a capture ELISA is designed to measure the amount of antibody present in a sample (typically a serological test), while a sandwich ELISA measures the amount of antigen in the sample. Thus, for a sandwich ELISA, a pair of antibodies to the target antigen is needed. The antigen is trapped between the capture antibody and the detector antibody (Fig. 1a). The example shown represents a direct binding sandwich ELISA since the detector antibody is directly labeled with an enzyme.

Robert Hnasko (ed.), *ELISA: Methods and Protocols*, Methods in Molecular Biology, vol. 1318,
DOI 10.1007/978-1-4939-2742-5_7, © Springer Science+Business Media New York 2015

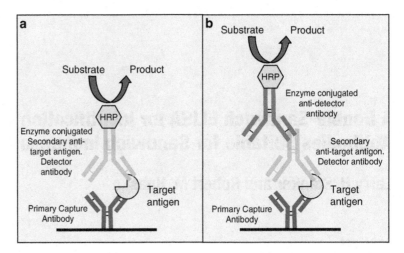

Fig. 1 Schematic of typical sandwich ELISAs. (**a**) Direct sandwich ELISA, (**b**) indirect sandwich ELISA

A common variant is the indirect sandwich ELISA (Fig. 1b) where the binding of the detector antibody is visualized by binding of a third antibody that is conjugated to the reporter molecule (i.e., if the detector antibody is made in a goat, the third or "reporter antibody" would be an enzyme-conjugated anti-goat antibody). In this scenario, the primary capture antibody could not be produced in goats but could be a mouse monoclonal antibody.

The detector and/or reporter antibody can be labeled with an enzyme and the sandwich detected with suitable colorimetric, fluorescent, or luminescent substrates. Alternatively, the detector antibody can be labeled with biotin and the sandwich detected using enzyme-conjugated streptavidin. The basic requirement of a sandwich ELISA (unless a repetitive epitope exists on the target antigen) is that two antibodies binding different epitopes on the same antigen are required. Furthermore, binding of one antibody must not interfere with binding of the second antibody even if they bind different epitopes.

Since the performance characteristics (specificity and sensitivity) of a sandwich ELISA are directly related to the quality of the antibodies (their binding affinities, stability, etc.). Finding matched antibody pairs, especially two monoclonal antibodies (mAbs), with these properties is often difficult. Monoclonal antibodies offer many advantages versus polyclonal antibodies including identification of the antibody-binding epitope, improved assay specificity and reliability since a positive result requires binding of two highly specific reagents with known epitopes, the ability to select high-affinity conformational antibodies with the desired binding specificity, and a consistent source of high-quality reagent. The sandwich ELISA itself has many advantages including that the sample need not be purified before analysis. Antigen purification and concentration is accomplished during the capture phase of the assay resulting in a three- to fivefold (or greater) increase in sensitivity versus a direct or indirect ELISA. Sandwich ELISAs usually display high specificity and greater confidence in the result because target detection requires binding of two distinct antibodies. However, their ability to detect low levels of target in complex samples makes them ideal tests for measuring the presence of the target antigen in unknown samples, e.g., food, environmental, or clinical samples.

Research in our laboratory has focused on development of sensitive immunoassays for botulinum neurotoxin (BoNT) [2–5]. Botulinum neurotoxins are produced by the anaerobic bacterium *Clostridium botulinum*. These toxins, as with many bacterial toxins, are large, complex di-chain protein toxins. In the case of BoNT, the active molecule consists of a 100 kDa heavy chain and a 50 kDa light chain joined by a single disulfide bond. Our initial approach was to screen hybridoma cell fusion supernatants using traditional indirect ELISA. Neurotoxin was adsorbed onto the bottoms of 96-well microassay plates. Supernatants from cell fusion experiments were added and antibody binding detected using an anti-mouse antibody conjugated to horseradish peroxidase (HRP). Earlier studies to develop monoclonal antibody-based sandwich ELISA for detecting BoNT serotype B [3] were only partially successful since the majority of the mAbs isolated failed to bind the toxin in solution. All of the mAbs isolated displayed strong binding in the indirect ELISA (impressive titration curves), good specificity (i.e., binding serotype B but not serotype A), and strong binding on Western blots. However, none of these antibodies bound the toxin in solution; hence, none were suitable as capture antibodies for a sandwich ELISA. A discouraging result after expending significant resources to generate the hybridoma clones, purify the mAbs and label with biotin in order to identify suitable antibody pairs for a sandwich ELISA. Adsorbing protein antigens onto the plastic surface of microassay wells can result in modifications of the protein. Many changes can be envisioned including changes to the surface charge of the protein, mild denaturation resulting in exposure of cryptic epitopes, and blocking surface epitopes [6]. Studies in our laboratory suggested that BoNT was modified when absorbed onto the plastic bottoms of microassay wells [3]. Similar results were observed with two different BoNT serotypes and with nontoxic BoNT-associated proteins. Interestingly, the BoNT antibodies could be induced to bind toxin in solution by treating the toxin with weak SDS solutions or adjusting the pH [3]. However, these steps necessitate additional sample preparation and only marginally improved assay performance. The double-capture ELISA outlined in Fig. 2 was applied as a screening tool to evaluate large numbers of hybridomas supernatants following cell fusion experiments in order to select for mAbs able to capture toxin in solution. Using this screen, it has been possible to select useful antibody pairs

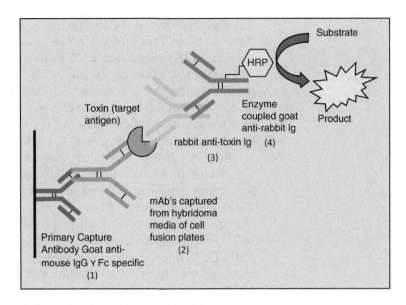

Fig. 2 The double-capture ELISA. The assay schematic shown here was used as the primary screen of cell fusion experiments to identify hybridomas that were producing antitoxin mAbs

and construct sandwich ELISAs for both BoNT serotypes B [6], E, and F (latter two unpublished) as well as good antibody pairs for the nontoxic BoNT hemagglutinin-70-associated protein [4].

Once mAbs suitable for a sandwich immunoassay are identified, they can be formatted into numerous different tests, e.g., sandwich ELISA, lateral-flow devices, and various immunobiosensors. The critical reagents in these different assay formats are the antibodies [7, 8].

2   Materials

Prepare all solutions using ultrapure water (prepared by reverse osmosis to attain a sensitivity of 18 MΩ at 22 °C). All reagents were stored at 4 °C (unless indicated) and warmed to room temperature before use. All studies involving animals followed protocols approved by the USDA Western Regional Research Center's Institutional Animal Care and Use Committee.

2.1 Double-Capture ELISA Components

1. Tris-buffered saline (TBS): 0.2 M Tris–HCl, 0.9 % NaCl, pH 7.4. Add 900 mL water to a 1-L bottle. Add 100 mL of a 10× Tris-buffered saline solution (Sigma-Aldrich T5912). Mix and store at 4 °C.

2. TBS containing 0.05 % Tween-20 (TBST). Adjust 0.5 mL of Tween-20 to 1 L with TBS.

3. 0.05 M carbonate buffer (pH 9.6). Dissolve one buffer capsule (Sigma #3041) in 100 mL water.

4. Blocking solution: 5 % powered nonfat milk (Carnation) in TBST. Store at 4 °C.

5. 96-well microassay plates (Immulon/Greiner/Nunc) (*see* **Note 1**).

2.2 Antigens and Conjugates

1. Affinity-purified goat anti-mouse immunoglobulin, Fc γ-specific fragment subclass I (Thermo Scientific # 31236, 1.2 mg/mL) (*see* **Note 2**).

2. Horseradish peroxidase (HRP) conjugated to goat anti-mouse immunoglobulin (whole molecule).

3. Streptavidin-HRP conjugate 1.25 mg/mL (Invitrogen 43-4323).

4. Affinity-purified, serotype-specific polyclonal rabbit anti-botulinum neurotoxin immunoglobulin (Metabiologics, Inc.)

5. HRP conjugated to goat anti-rabbit immunoglobulin (whole molecule) (Sigma # A6154).

2.3 Substrates

1. SuperSignal ELISA Femto maximum sensitivity luminescent substrate (Thermo Scientific #37074).

2. SuperSignal West Pico chemiluminescent substrate (Thermo Scientific #34078) (*see* **Note 3**).

3 Methods

All procedures are carried out at room temperature unless otherwise indicated. Preparation of BoNT dilutions, additions to assay plates, and plate washing performed in a biosafety cabinet (BSC) (Class 2 B2).

3.1 Preparation of 96-Well Microassay Plates

1. Prepare primary capture antibody-coated microassay plates as follows. Add 100 μL/well of a 1 μg/mL solution of goat anti-mouse IgG Fc γ fragment (Thermo Scientific #31236) prepared in 0.05 M carbonate buffer (pH 9.6) to black, flat-bottom, Maxisorp 96-well microassay plates (Nunc). Cover the plates with 96-well plate lids or plastic film sheets. Incubate the plates at 4 °C overnight or until needed (*see* **Notes 4** and **2**).

2. Aspirate the primary capture antibody solution and block remaining reactive sites by adding 300 μL per well of a solution of 5 % nonfat dry milk prepared in TBST buffer. Cover the plate and incubate at 37 °C for 1 h (*see* **Note 5**).

3. Aspirate the block solution and add 100 μL (as little as 50 μL can be used) per well of hybridoma supernatant obtained from 96-well cell culture plates following a cell fusion experiment.

The plates are then covered and incubated at 37 °C for 1 h (*see* **Note 6**).

4. The hybridoma supernatant is aspirated and the plates washed three times with TBST using an automatic plate washer (BioTek ELx405 Select plate washer) (*see* **Note 7**).

5. Add antigen to the plate. For BoNT, we add 50 μL of a 200 ng/mL solution in blocking buffer. The plates are then sealed with adhesive plastic film, placed in a secondary containment tray, and incubated 1 h at 37 °C (*see* **Note 8**).

6. The plates are next washed a minimum of three times with TBST buffer using an ELx405 plate washer in a BSC.

7. Next 50 μL of the secondary detection antibody, in this example a rabbit polyclonal anti-BoNT (Metabiologics, Inc.) diluted 1:5,000 (when the stock solution is at 1 mg/mL), is added to the plates. The plates are sealed with plastic films and incubated at 37 °C.

8. The plates are then washed as in **step 6** above.

9. Next 50 μL of a 1–5,000 dilution of an HRP-conjugated goat anti-rabbit IgG (whole molecule), affinity (isolated, antigen-specific antibody (Sigma # A6154) is added to each well. The plates are then covered and incubated at 37 °C for 1 h.

10. The plates are then washed a total of 6 times with TBST as in **step 6** above.

11. For evaluation of primary cell fusion plates, 50 μL SuperSignal West Pico chemiluminescent substrate (Thermo scientific #34078) prepared as suggested by the manufacturer (equal parts of the A and B solution are mixed immediately before use) is added to the plates. The plates are then incubated at room temperature with shaking for 3 min. The luminescent signal is recorded with a 96-well plate luminescence reader (PerkinElmer #2030 VICTOR X^3 Multilabel Plate Reader or a Berthold LB962 CentroPRO Luminescence Microplate Reader) set for 0.1 s per well. Data is captured and analyzed with Excel (Microsoft) (*see* **Note 9**). Results from a typical double-capture ELISA screen of 96-well hybridoma cell culture plates are shown in Fig. 3.

4   Notes

1. We generally use black 96-well plates for our luminescent assays even though white plates are recommended generally for luminescence and black plates for fluorescence. We find that white plates result in a higher background signal and consistently use black plates. We have used plates from various manufacturers with differences noted in assay performance.

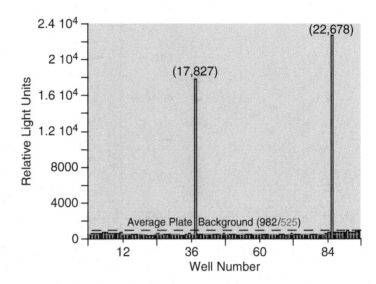

Fig. 3 Results from a typical double-capture ELISA screen of 96-well cell fusion plates. The dashed red line represents the background activity of the plate minus the two obvious positive wells (525 counts). Often we simply calculate the average activity based on all 96-wells (*black dashed line* 982 counts). The two positive wells regardless of the calculation of background are readily detected

2. Since multiple antibodies are used in the double-capture ELISA, it is critical that these be evaluated for nonspecific cross-reactivity. In the example described here, we find that the goat anti-mouse Ig capture antibody and the rabbit antitoxin antibody were the most problematic. Shown in Fig. 4 is a simple titration demonstrating the cross-reactivity of four, affinity-purified, goat anti-mouse commercial antibodies with the rabbit anti-BoNT serotype B antibody. In our screening assay, we use the rabbit antitoxin antibody at a concentration of 1 μg/mL. Clearly, the antibody from sources #1 and #4 resulted in excess signal and would be unsuitable or use in this assay. In contrast, the anti-mouse antibodies from either source #2 or #3 reacted minimally with the rabbit antitoxin. We found that little cross-reactivity occurred between the HRP goat anti-rabbit antibody and the goat anti-mouse antibody.

3. For routine double-capture ELISA screens of fusion wells and general antibody characterization, we use the SuperSignal West Pico substrate. After suitable antibody pairs are identified, we use the SuperSignal ELISA Femto substrate. Significantly higher counts are obtained with the Femto substrate resulting in more sensitive assays. If the highest degree of sensitivity is necessary to screen cell fusion plates, I suggest the use of the Femto substrate.

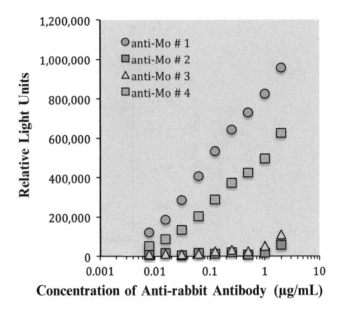

Fig. 4 ELISA titration demonstrating the reactivity of goat anti-Mo IgG from different manufacturers with the anti-BoNT/F generated in rabbit. The goat anti-mouse was absorbed onto the plates (100 μL of a 1 μg/mL solution), the plates blocked, the rabbit antitoxin added at the concentrations indicated followed by HRP-conjugated anti-rabbit antibody. Earlier studies demonstrated no cross-reactivity between the HRP conjugate and the goat anti-mouse antibody

4. A variety of 96-well microliter plates can be used. Plates from different manufacturers, i.e., Immulon and Greiner, performed satisfactorily in our experiments. As little as 50 μL per well can be used; black or clear plates work best. White plates exhibited a pronounced edge effect and higher background signals.

5. During reagent addition and washing of the 96-well assay plates, it is necessary to take care that the pipette tips or pins of an automatic plate washer do not come in contact with the bottoms of the wells. This leads to scratching of the plate bottom resulting in exposure of non-blocked surfaces, ultimately resulting in higher backgrounds.

6. Cells can be removed from the hybridoma supernatants by centrifugation although this does not appear to improve assay performance or decreasing background. Careful pipetting of 50–100 μL from the upper level of the cell culture plate works well. If we transfer the hybridoma supernatant manually with a 12-channel pipette, we transfer the supernatants into sterile 96-well microculture plates in order to maintain the sterility of the cell fusion plates. Often we use a 96-well transfer system (TranStar) in which case we transfer directly from the hybridoma plates into the blocked assay plates. Sterility is maintained since the tips of the transfer cartridges do not touch the assay

plates. When using the TranStar system, we do not change cartridges between plates even though there is some supernatant carryover. The major advantage of not changing cartridges is the speed of transferring the sample from all of the cell fusion plates. A disadvantage is that there is a small amount of media carryover that can result in a highly positive well remaining positive for the next one or two transfers. This is easily seen when evaluating the screening results.

7. Plate washing is a critical step in the assay and is greatly facilitated by use of a multiwell automatic plate washer. Ensure that the washing pins are adjusted for the specific 96-well plates being used, paying particular attention to adjusting the washing pin depth in order to avoid contact with the plate bottom. Wash a minimum of three times. Additional washings often improve background levels.

8. An obviously critical step is the choice of antigen. Since we are interested in developing test to measure toxin, we use intact, non-denatured toxin in order to identify hybridoma antibodies that can capture the toxin out of solution under physiological conditions. The use of toxin at this step is possible since anti-toxin antiserum was available for the subsequent steps in the assay. In other studies, we immunized with recombinant GST-antigen polypeptide fragments. If no appropriate detector antibody existed, we measured the ability of the monoclonal antibodies to capture the recombinant GST-toxin fragment by probing with an antibody to GST. Again, it is critical to evaluate different sources of anti-GST and anti-mouse Ig in order to minimize background. For some projects, we already have at least one monoclonal antibody capable of acting as a detector antibody. Thus, it was relatively simple to purify and biotin label this mAb and use it as the detector antibody. In some experiments where no detector antibody reagents were available, we labeled the antigen directly with biotin. In all of these examples, we used streptavidin-HRP. All manipulations using BoNT were carried out in a biological safety cabinet.

9. The SuperSignal West Pico substrate was routinely used. If more sensitivity is desired, the SuperSignal ELISA Femto substrate can be substituted.

References

1. Engvall E, Perlmann P (1971) Enzyme-linked immunosorbent assay (ELISA) quantitative assay of immunoglobulin G. Immunochemistry 8:871–874

2. Stanker LH, Merrill P, Scotcher MC et al (2008) Development and partial characterization of high-affinity monoclonal antibodies for botulinum toxin type A and their use in analysis of milk by sandwich ELISA. J Immunol Methods 336:1–8

3. Scotcher MC, Cheng LW, Stanker LH (2010) Detection of botulinum neurotoxin serotype B

at sub mouse LD50 levels by a sandwich immunoassay and its application to toxin detection in milk. PLoS One 5:e11047

4. Scotcher M, Chen L, Ching K et al (2013) Development and characterization of six monoclonal antibodies to hemagglutinin-70 (HA70) of Clostridium botulinum and their application in a sandwich ELISA. Monoclon Antib Immunodiagn Immunother 32:6–15

5. He J (2013) Practical guide to ELISA development. In: David G (ed) The immunoassay handbook, 4th edn. Wild, Elsevier Ltd, Amsterdam, The Netherlands, pp 381–395. ISBN 978-0-08-097037-0

6. Cheng L, Stanker LH (2013) Detection of botulinum neurotoxin serotypes A and B using chemiluminescence and electrochemiluminescence immunoassays in food and serum matrices. J Agric Food Chem 61:755–760

7. Ching KH, Lin A, McGarvey JA et al (2012) Rapid and selective detection of botulinum neurotoxin serotype-A and –B with a single immunochromatographic test strip. J Immunol Methods 380:23–29

8. Stanker LH, Scotcher MC, Cheng L et al (2013) A monoclonal antibody based capture ELISA for botulinum neurotoxin serotype B: toxin detection in Food. Toxins 5:2212–2226

Chapter 8

ELISpot and DC-ELISpot Assay to Measure Frequency of Antigen-Specific IFNγ-Secreting Cells

Marcelo A. Navarrete

Abstract

ELISpot is a highly sensitive method in immunology to enumerate cells producing a given cytokine. Cells are stimulated in a microtiter plate pre-coated with a specific anti-analyte antibody. In response to the stimulation, cells release cytokines that are bound to the anti-analyte antibody. After a washing step, which removes the cells from the wells, the location of the cytokine-releasing cell is visualized by an enzyme-labeled detection antibody and its corresponding chromogenic substrate. The end result is a set of colored spots, each of which represents an area where a cell secreting the cytokine had been located.

Here we describe the standard ELISpot protocol and a variation denominated dendritic cell (DC)-ELISpot for the detection of IFNγ-secreting cells upon stimulation with oligopeptides and protein antigens, respectively.

Key words ELISpot, Dendritic cell, T-cell frequency, Immune response, Antigen

1   Introduction

The enzyme-linked immunosorbent spot (ELISpot) assay is an ELISA-based method commonly used for the identification and enumeration of cytokine-producing cells with exquisite sensitivity at the single-cell level [1].

One of the most common applications of the assay is the enumeration of IFNγ-secreting cells in response to antigenic stimulation. Typically, the assay is performed by stimulating antigen-specific T cells within peripheral blood mononuclear cells (PBMCs) in wells coated with an antibody that binds to the desired cytokine. In response to the recognition of the antigen, T cells specifically release IFNγ, which is then trapped to the anti-IFNγ antibody. After a washing step, which removes the cells from the wells, the location of the cytokine-releasing cell is visualized by an enzyme-labeled detection antibody and its corresponding chromogenic substrate, which has to be non-soluble to become attached to the surface of a well. The end result is a set of colored spots,

Robert Hnasko (ed.), *ELISA: Methods and Protocols*, Methods in Molecular Biology, vol. 1318,
DOI 10.1007/978-1-4939-2742-5_8, © Springer Science+Business Media New York 2015

each of which represents an area where a cell secreting IFNγ had been located.

T cells present among the PBMC recognize peptides presented on the HLA surface of antigen-presenting cells (APC) like monocytes and macrophages also present in the PBMC sample. Whereas HLA-binding oligopeptides can be added directly to the ELISpot assay without the necessity of a preincubation step, complex protein antigens must be internalized and processed by professional antigen-presenting cells (APC) for efficient presentation via HLA class I or II [2, 3]. To overcome this issue, we have developed a serum-free DC-ELISpot protocol using standardized DC for sensitive enumeration of T cells recognizing protein antigens, based on the assay described by Nehete and colleagues [4, 5]. In this variation of the ELISpot assay, the stimulation is performed with autologous DC previously loaded with the desired protein antigen.

Here we describe the standard and the DC-ELISpot assay protocol for the detection of IFNγ-secreting cells upon antigen stimulation. For measuring immune responses against oligopeptide antigens, a direct ELISpot protocol may be used; however, when the target antigen is a protein, the DC-ELISpot should be the preferred protocol. Figure 1 summarizes the steps of the assay.

Although the assay is described to detect IFNγ-secreting cells, it can be easily adapted for the detection of other cytokines providing that the appropriate capture and detection antibody pair is available.

2 Materials

Prepare all solutions under sterile conditions; use cell culture-grade and analytical-grade reagents as required. Prepare and store all reagents at 4 °C (unless otherwise indicated). Diligently follow all waste disposal regulations when disposing waste materials. Avoid the use of sodium azide.

Cell Culture Reagents

1. Serum-free ELISpot cell culture medium: CellGro DC Medium (CellGenix, Freiburg, Germany) supplemented with penicillin/streptomycin. Keep sterile and store at 4 °C.

2. PMA/ionomycin solution: requires phorbol 12-myristate 13-acetate (PMA, cell culture grade, Sigma-Aldrich) and ionomycin (cell culture grade, Sigma-Aldrich). Prepare a fresh solution containing 10 ng/ml PMA and 4 μg/ml ionomycin in the ELISpot cell culture medium.

ELISpot Assay Reagents

3. Dulbecco's phosphate-buffered saline (DPBS) without calcium and magnesium. Keep sterile and store at room temperature.

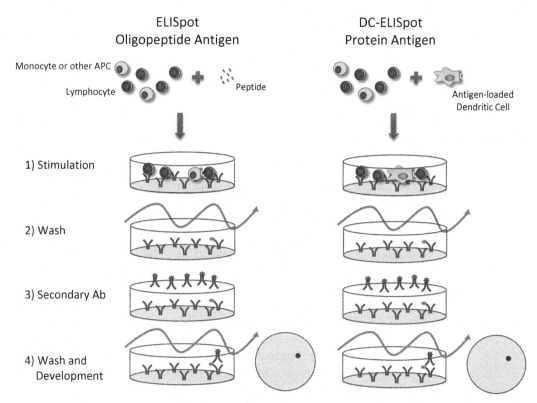

Fig. 1 Schematic overview of the ELISpot assay (*left*) and the DC-ELISpot variation (*right*). In the standard protocol, peripheral blood mononuclear cell (PBMC) sample is incubated in the presence of oligopeptides that bound to the HLA surface of antigen-presenting cells (APC) present among the PBMC. If the antigen is a protein, the antigen needs to be processed and presented by professional APC. Since dendritic cells are the most potent type of APC, the DC-ELISpot is the preferred protocol for the measurement of immune response against protein antigens

4. Serum-free ELISpot medium: CellGro DC Medium (CellGenix, Freiburg, Germany) supplemented with penicillin/streptomycin. Keep sterile and store at 4 °C.

5. 96-well MultiScreen plate, hydrophobic with PVDF membrane.

6. Human IFNγ ELISpot pair (recommended: BD™ ELISpot catalog #551873).

7. ELISpot washing buffer: DPBS containing 0.005 % Tween 20.

8. Streptavidin-alkaline phosphatase enzyme conjugate, 1:1,000 dilution in DPBS (recommended: Bio-Rad, #170-3554).

9. AP Conjugate Substrate Kit (recommended: Bio-Rad, #170-6432).

10. Dilute 25× AP color development buffer 1:25 in water (400 μl AP + 9,600 μl H₂O). Buffer can be distributed in aliquots and stored at 4 °C.

Equipment

11. Laminar flow cabinet.

12. CO_2 cell culture incubator.

13. Automated ELISpot reader.

---

3   Methods

This assay makes use of life cells; therefore, the processing of samples and/or performing cell culture-based assays on clinical specimens from patients and animals must be performed in the appropriate biosafety level (BSL) laboratory (BSL-2 or above depending on the type of sample). Laboratory safety procedures include at least all standard BSL-2 procedures with enhancements as follows: (1) laboratory personnel have specific training in handling pathogenic and potentially lethal agents and are supervised by competent scientists who are experienced in working with these agents; and (2) the laboratory should have special engineering and design features to ensure directional airflow from clean to potentially contaminated areas. Supervisors are responsible for ensuring that technicians are properly trained to work safely in the laboratory.

3.1   Coat Primary Antibody (Day 1)

1. Pre-wet each well of a 96-well MultiScreen plate (hydrophobic with PVDF membrane) with 15 µl of 35 % ethanol in sterile water for 1 min. Rinse with 150 µl sterile DPBS three times before the ethanol evaporates (*see* **Note 1**).

2. Dilute 50 µl purified anti-IFNγ in 5 ml sterile PBS (15 µg/ml). Coat MultiScreen plates with 50 µl/well. Incubate overnight at 4 °C (*see* **Note 2**).

3.2   Preparation of PBMCs and DC for ELISpot Assay (Day 1)

All these steps must be performed under sterile conditions in a laminar flow cabinet. Keep the cells on ice during preparation to prevent unspecific activation.

1. The PBMC sample can be obtained from a fresh gradient centrifugation or a previously frozen sample stored in vapor phase of liquid nitrogen. If protein antigens need to be measured, prepare dendritic cells (DC) under serum-free condition and load the DC with the desired antigen as previously described [4, 6, 7].

   When working with frozen samples, it is recommended to rest the cells overnight in serum-free ELISpot cell culture medium for at least 4 h [8] as follows.

2. Resuspend the cells in serum-free ELISpot medium at a concentration of 4×10^6 cells/ml and plate 5 ml of the suspension into each well of a 6-well plate.

3. Rest at least 4 h or overnight in a cell culture incubator at 37 °C, 5 % CO_2.

4. Harvest the cells: transfer pipette the content of a well in a 15 ml Falcon tube. Pellet the cells by centrifuging 8 min at $300 \times g$ at 4 °C.

5. Resuspend the cell pellet adjusting the cell count at 4×10^6 viable cells/ml in serum-free ELISpot medium (you will need 100 μl of this suspension per well of the ELISpot plate). Cell viability should be higher than 80 % (more than 90 % is recommended). Keep the cells on ice until transfer to the ELISpot plate (*see* **Note 3**).

3.3 Stimulation (Day 1)

All these steps must be performed under sterile conditions in a laminar flow cabinet.

Block Membrane with Serum-Free ELISpot Medium

1. Decant primary antibody solution.

2. Wash off unbound antibody with 150 μl sterile DPBS, decant wash, and repeat.

3. Block membrane with 150 μl/well of serum-free ELISpot medium for at least 2 h at 37 °C.

Cell Culture and Stimulation

4. Stimulation: Plate 100 μl/well of the rested PBMC suspension ($1–4 \times 10^6$ viable cells/ml = $1–4 \times 10^5$ viable cells/well) together with 100 μl/well of the peptide diluted in serum-free ELISpot medium at a concentration of 1–10 μg/ml in at least three replicates. If the stimulator is a protein, add instead 100 μl/well of antigen-loaded DC suspension ($1–10 \times 10^4$ viable cells/ml = $1–10 \times 10^3$ viable cells/well) (*see* **Notes 4** and **5**).

5. Background control: Plate 100 μl/well of the rested PBMC suspension ($1–4 \times 10^6$ viable cells/ml = $1–4 \times 10^5$ viable cells/well) together with 100 μl/well of serum-free ELISpot medium. If the stimulator is a protein, add instead 100 μl/well of non-loaded DC suspension ($1–10 \times 10^4$ viable cells/ml = $1–10 \times 10^3$ viable cells/well).

6. As positive control, plate 10×10^3 PBMC/well triplicate in 150 μl ELISpot-incubation medium + 50 μl PMA/ionomycin solution.

7. Incubate overnight at 37 °C 5 % CO_2.
Important: Do not disturb the plate during the incubation period or artifacts may form.

3.4 Secondary Antibody and Detection (Day 2)

The following steps do not require sterile conditions. Use appropriate BSL-2 biosafety procedures.

Secondary Antibody

1. Flick and blot to decant cells (*see* **Note 6**).

2. Wash the plate six times with ELISpot washing buffer. *Important*: The ELISpot washing buffer is DPBS with 0.005 % Tween 20. It is important not to exceed 0.01 % Tween 20 to prevent the possibility of leakage and artifacts.

3. Dilute 2 μg/ml biotinylated anti-IFNγ antibody in DPBS/0.5 % human serum albumin and add 100 μl/well.

4. Incubate for 30 min at 37 °C, 5 % CO_2, and 95 % humidity (or alternatively at 4 °C overnight).

5. Wash the plate six times with ELISpot washing buffer.

Enzyme Conjugate and Substrate Development

6. Prepare streptavidin-alkaline phosphatase enzyme conjugate at 1:1,000 dilution in DPBS.

7. Add 100 μl per well of the diluted streptavidin-alkaline phosphatase. Incubate for 30 min at room temperature in the dark (cover the plate with aluminum foil) (*see* **Note 7**).

8. Decant streptavidin, and wash three times with ELISpot washing buffer, followed by four washes with DPBS without Tween 20 (*see* **Note 8**).

9. Dilute 25× AP color development buffer 1:25 in water (400 μl AP + 9,600 μl H_2O).

10. Add 100 μl of reagent A and 100 μl of reagent B to 10 ml of the previous solution.

11. Add 100 μl/well of development solution.

12. Incubate in the dark until it is possible to see the spots in the positive control wells for 7–10 min (*see* **Note 9**).

13. Stop development under running water and wash extensively. While washing, remove the underdrain and continue rinsing.

14. Let plate dry in the dark.

Plate Reading

15. Read the plates in an automated ELISpot reader; the reading process is performed in a semiautomated process. Trained personnel should make adequate adjustments for technical artifacts and audit the read process. For data analysis and positivity criteria, we recommend to refer to Moodie et al. [9].

4   Notes

1. Once the membrane is pre-wet with alcohol, do not allow the membrane to dry for the duration of the assay. Make sure that the selected plate is compatible with your ELISpot reader.

2. Plates coated with the anti-analyte antibody can be stored at 4 °C up to 4 weeks. Seal the plates with Parafilm to avoid leakage and prevent evaporation.

3. High cell viability is required for sensitive and accurate frequency estimation. Low viability may lead to unspecific background and underestimation of the real frequency of the cytokine-releasing cells. However, if only a sample with low viability is available, acceptable results can be achieved by depletion of dead cells with the Miltenyi Biotec Dead Cell Removal Kit immediately before plating.

4. Triplicate is the minimum number of required replicates in the sample and the background control. The use of four replicates or more is recommended.

5. In the DC-ELISpot protocol, the number of cells and the PBMC/DC ratio need to be established and carefully titrated for each individual application and/or protein type. As a guide, 400,000 PBMC/well with 4,000 DC/well can be used as a starting point.

6. In certain experimental setups, the measurement of cytokines in the supernatant may be of interest. When removing the supernatant, avoid contact of the pipette tip with the filter that may result in artifact formation.

7. This step is critical and exceeding 1 h incubation with enzyme conjugate will result in increased background color.

8. The final washes with DPBS are important as Tween 20 will interfere with the spot development. If you observe weak or fuzzy spots, increase the number of washing steps at this point.

9. The moment to stop development is critical for an adequate visualization of the spots. Spots in positive control wells are normally the first to be visualized. Once you observe spot formation in these wells, proceed to stop immediately regardless of the apparition of spots in other wells. Other spots will be clearly visualized after the plate dried out.

References

1. Czerkinsky CC, Nilsson LA, Nygren H et al (1983) A solid-phase enzyme-linked immunospot (ELISPOT) assay for enumeration of specific antibody-secreting cells. J Immunol Methods 65:109–121

2. Keilholz U, Weber J, Finke JH et al (2002) Immunologic monitoring of cancer vaccine therapy: results of a workshop sponsored by the Society for Biological Therapy. J Immunother 25:97–138

3. Scheibenbogen C, Lee KH, Mayer S et al (1997) A sensitive ELISPOT assay for detection of CD8+ T lymphocytes specific for HLA class I-binding peptide epitopes derived from influenza proteins in the blood of healthy donors and melanoma patients. Clin Cancer Res 3:221–226

4. Navarrete MA, Bertinetti-Lapatki C, Michelfelder I et al (2013) Usage of standardized antigen-presenting cells improves ELISpot performance for complex protein antigens. J Immunol Methods 391:146–153

5. Nehete PN, Gambhira R, Nehete BP et al (2003) Dendritic cells enhance detection of antigen-specific cellular immune responses by lymphocytes from rhesus macaques immunized with an HIV envelope peptide cocktail vaccine. J Med Primatol 32:67–73

6. Moller I, Michel K, Frech N et al (2008) Dendritic cell maturation with poly(I:C)-based versus PGE2-based cytokine combinations results in differential functional characteristics relevant to clinical application. J Immunother 31:506–519

7. Warncke M, Dodero A, Dierbach H et al (2006) Murine dendritic cells generated under serum-free conditions have a mature phenotype and efficiently induce primary immune responses. J Immunol Methods 310:1–11

8. Malyguine A, Strobl SL, Shafer-Weaver KA et al (2004) A modified human ELISPOT assay to detect specific responses to primary tumor cell targets. J Transl Med 2:9

9. Moodie Z, Price L, Gouttefangeas C et al (2010) Response definition criteria for ELISPOT assays revisited. Cancer Immunol Immunother 59: 1489–1501

Chapter 9

The Western Blot

Thomas S. Hnasko and Robert M. Hnasko

Abstract

Western blotting is a technique that involves the separation of proteins by gel electrophoresis, their blotting or transfer to a membrane, and selective immunodetection of an immobilized antigen. This is an important and routine method for protein analysis that depends on the specificity of antibody-antigen interaction and is useful for the qualitative or semiquantitative identification of specific proteins and their molecular weight from a complex mixture. This chapter will outline the requisite steps including gel electrophoresis of a protein sample, transfer of protein from a gel to a membrane support, and immunodetection of a target antigen.

Key words Western blot, Immunoblot, Enzyme-linked immunodetection, SDS-PAGE, Gel electrophoresis

1 Introduction

Western blotting or immunoblotting refers to the separation of proteins by polyacrylamide gel electrophoresis (PAGE) based on size, their subsequent transfer and immobilization to a membrane support, and their selective detection using an antibody-mediated reporter system [1]. This technique is routinely used to qualitatively identify a specific protein from a complex biological sample and provide information about its molecular weight.

The first step is sample preparation that requires the solubilization of the proteins in a lysis buffer, often containing protease inhibitors and detergents [2, 3] (*see* **Note 1**). Accurate determination of protein concentration, for example, using bicinchoninic acid (BCA) or Bradford assays (*see* **Note 2**), is important as polyacrylamide gels have a limited protein load capacity to achieve adequate molecular weight separation [4, 5].

The soluble protein sample is diluted with a sample loading buffer concentrate that contains an indicator dye such as bromophenol blue, the anionic denaturing detergent sodium dodecyl sulfate (SDS), and glycerol. The loading sample can then be denatured

Robert Hnasko (ed.), *ELISA: Methods and Protocols*, Methods in Molecular Biology, vol. 1318,
DOI 10.1007/978-1-4939-2742-5_9, © Springer Science+Business Media New York 2015

by heating for 5–10 min between 70 and 100 °C. This process unfolds the proteins causing the loss of secondary conformational structures (*see* **Note 3**) and surrounds them with SDS molecules that impart a negative charge so that all proteins migrate toward the positive pole during PAGE. Prior to heat denaturation, a chemical-reducing agent, such as dithiothreitol (DTT) or 2-mercaptoethanol, can be added to the sample to disrupt intra- and inter-chain disulfide bonds further unfolding complex secondary and tertiary protein structures (*see* **Note 4**).

The percentage of polyacrylamide used in the gel along with the buffer system will influence the mobility of the proteins through the gel as current is applied. The expected size of the target protein can be used to select the best gel/buffer system to achieve optimal separation and resolution (*see* Fig. 1). The prepared protein samples are loaded into wells of the gel aided by the dye indicator and glycerol in the sample loading buffer, current is applied, and proteins migrate through the gel (*see* Fig. 2) and are separated by charge (which is proportional to size). A protein standard composed of a pool of proteins of known molecular weights is included in one well/lane. We prefer color protein standards as they visually separate in the gel during electrophoresis and provide a measure of distance traveled, the degree of separation, and a visual metric for the efficacy of protein transfer to membrane [6].

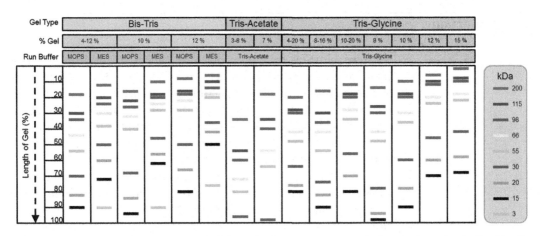

Fig. 1 Migration of protein by molecular weight varies by gel type, concentration, and running buffer. Use the estimated migration patterns provided here to assist in the selection of gel type and running buffer based on the predicted MW of the target protein and the desired separation

Fig. 2 (continued) in place, and fill reservoirs with running buffer. Use a P200 pipette with gel-loading tip and carefully rinse wells with running buffer. (**c**) Load samples containing indicator dye into wells. (**d**) Apply lid, turn on power supply, and monitor progress by visualization of indicator dye. (*1*) NuPAGE precast gel, (*2*) extracted disposable comb, (*3*) sealing tape, (*4*) gel knife for extracting and trimming gel following the run, (*5*) cassette base, (*6*) clamp to tighten gel cassettes against rubber seal of cassette base, (*7*) upper reservoir, (*8*) lower reservoir, (*9*) sample wells, (*10*) tank lid, (*11*) dye indicator nearing end of run

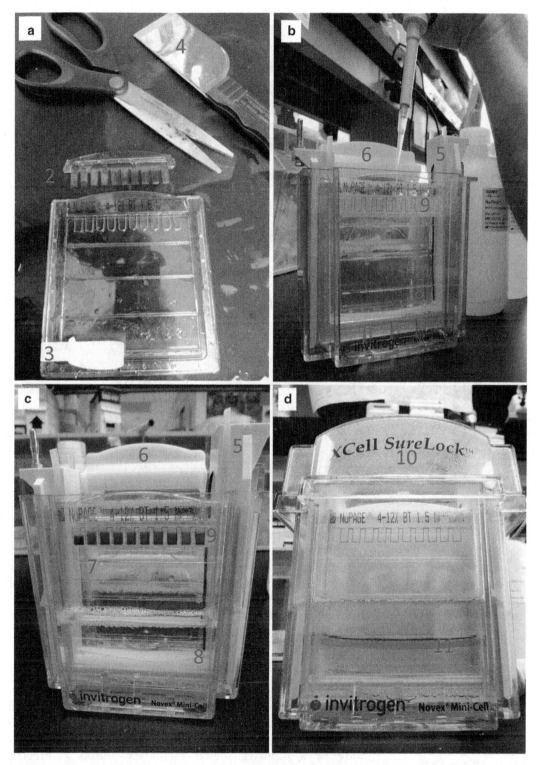

Fig. 2 Setting up polyacrylamide gel electrophoresis (PAGE). (**a**) Carefully extract comb from the top of the precast NuPAGE gel and remove tape from the bottom. (**b**) Assemble the tank by placing gel cassettes ($n = 2$) back-to-back against the rubber seals of the cassette base to create a tight upper and lower reservoir, clamp

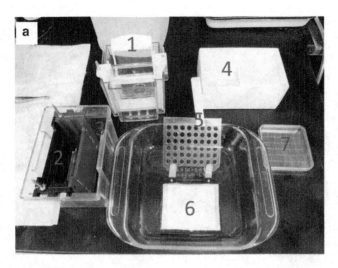

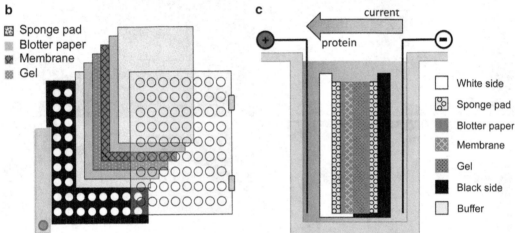

Fig. 3 Assembling gel for transfer to nitrocellulose membrane. (**a**) Following the completion of PAGE, assemble materials required for the transfer of protein from gel to membrane. (**b**) Schematic illustration of the sequence of blot components in the transfer cassette. (**c**) Schematic illustration of the orientation of blot components within the cassette in transfer tank and the direction of the current flow. Note that the membrane must be between the gel and the positive (*red*) pole of the transfer box. (*1*) Gel in runner tank following PAGE, (*2*) buffer tank and cassette holder, (*3*) space for ice cooling brick, (*4*) precut nitrocellulose and blotting paper, (*5*) Mini-Trans-Blot cassette, (*6*) sponge assembly, (*7*) square plastic dish for pre-wetting blot paper, (*8*) glass Pyrex dish for submersion assembling of blot components

The gel-separated proteins are transferred and immobilized to a nitrocellulose or polyvinylidene fluoride (PVDF) membrane (*see* Fig. 3). The membranes are washed, blocked, and incubated with analyte-specific primary antibody [6, 7]. Two common approaches include the use of a direct reporter-labeled primary antibody or a reporter-labeled secondary antibody directed against the host species of the primary antibody. The reporter conjugated to the antibody can be varied such as an enzyme that produces a color reaction product or luminescent signal at the site of antigen-antibody binding when exposed to a substrate or a direct fluorescent signal that is generated by excitation at a specific wavelength [8–10] (*see* **Note 5**). A detection system appropriate for the signal generated is necessary and some means of recording the results [11].

2   Materials

2.1   Protein Separation by Polyacrylamide Gel Electrophoresis (PAGE)

1. Xcell SureLock or blot (Invitrogen) that includes tank base, gel runner tank, tank lid, and cassette clamps.
2. Basic power supply with power pack adaptor cords (Bio-Rad).
3. Precast gel (NuPAGE) (*see* **Note 6**).
4. 20× 2-(N-morpholino)ethanesulfonic acid (MES) or 3-(N-morpholino)propanesulfonic acid (MOPS) running buffer (Invitrogen).
5. 4× lithium dodecyl sulfate (LDS) sample buffer (Invitrogen).
6. Heating block and timer.
7. Pipette and long narrow gel-loading tips.
8. 10× sample reducing buffer (Invitrogen).
9. Pre-stained protein ladder (250–2 kDa Dual Xtra; Bio-RAD).

2.2   Transfer of Protein from Gel to Membrane

1. Mini-Trans-Blot (Bio-Rad) that includes a tank, lid, and Mini-Trans-Blot module (two gel holder cassettes, foam pads, electrode assembly, and cooling unit). Store cooling ice brick in freezer so it is frozen when needed.
2. 0.45 μm nitrocellulose filter paper sandwiches 7×8.5 cm (Bio-Rad) (*see* **Note 7**).
3. 20× NuPAGE transfer buffer.
4. Methanol.
5. Square Pyrex dish.
6. Square disposable plastic 100×15 mm petri dish (Falcon).
7. Razor blade and gel knife.
8. Basic power supply with power pack adaptor cords (Bio-Rad).

2.3   Western Immunoblotting

1. 10× Tris-buffered saline with 1 % Tween 20 (TBST).
2. Shaker/agitator (Belly Dancer, Stovall).
3. 10 % powdered nonfat dry milk in TBST (Carnation).
4. Square disposable plastic 100×15 mm petri dish (Falcon).
5. Plastic pouches (Ampac tubular rollstock).
6. Impulse heat sealer (Cole-Parmer).
7. Primary antibody.

8. Secondary antibody conjugated to horseradish peroxidase (HRP) generated against host species of primary antibody (Thermo-Pierce).

9. SuperSignal enhanced chemiluminescent substrate (picoECL, Thermo-Pierce).

10. Gel documentation system (Alpha Innotech).

3 Methods

3.1 Polyacrylamide Gel Electrophoresis (PAGE)

1. Dilute the protein sample (4:1) in 4× LDS sample buffer to yield a 35 µg/mL 1× LDS protein solution, and vortex and heat at 70 °C for 10 min.

2. Centrifuge the sample briefly at $5,000 \times g$.

3. Prepare 1 L MES or MOPS running buffer by diluting 20× to 1× in ddH$_2$O.

4. Prepare precast gel by removing from storage pouch, gently remove well comb, and remove tape from the bottom of the plastic gel case (*see* Fig. 2a).

5. Place gel cassette in buffer tank against the rubber seal with the opening of the gel wells facing the inside of the upper tank reservoir. Ensure a tight fit to create a separate upper and lower buffer reservoir as the current will flow through the gel from the top to the slit at the bottom of the plastic gel cassette. This tank system is designed to run two gels simultaneously so if only running one, use a "dummy" cassette on the other side to create an upper reservoir.

6. Pour the running buffer into the upper reservoir and ensure no buffer leakage to the lower tank; pour the remaining buffer in the lower tank halfway, keeping the liquid below the upper reservoir.

7. Using the liquid from the upper reservoir with a P200 pipette and gel-loading tip, rinse each well to remove the storage glycerol and preservative. Take care to avoid puncturing the bottom of the well or disturbing the thin well sides (*see* Fig. 2b).

8. Load each well with equal volume of heat-denatured 1× LDS sample and reserve one lane for a protein ladder (*see* Fig. 2c) (*see* **Note 8**).

9. Place on lid and attach red and black cables to power supply.

10. Turn on power supply, run the gel at 200 V constant for 50 min, and note the movement of the indicator dye with time (*see* Fig. 2d) (*see* **Note 9**).

3.2 Transfer of Protein from Gel to Membrane

1. Prepare 1 L of 1× transfer buffer with 10 % methanol by diluting 20× stock (50 mL 20× stock, 100 mL methanol, 850 mL ddH$_2$O).

2. Place a gel knife between the plastic plates of the gel cassette and twist to open the plates. Remove one faceplate and trim with a razor blade the top of the gel from the bottom of the wells to create a straight line. Do the same at the bottom of the gel trimming away the excess gel "L" to create a flat horizontal line.

3. Using a square Pyrex dish, lay out the plastic transfer cassette with the black side down and cover with 1× transfer buffer. Soak two foam sponges, lay one on the black side, and lay down a filter paper on top of the foam making sure both are wet and slightly submerged. Gently place the gel down on the wet filter paper with the top of the gel oriented to the top of the transfer cassette closure (*see* Fig. 3a). Wet the cut nitrocellulose membrane with 1× transfer buffer making sure it is completely wet (with even appearance) by rocking. While submerged, place the nitrocellulose on top of the gel making sure there are no bubbles between the gel and the membrane, hold in place, add wet filter paper, and then foam sponge to create the sandwich all while submerged in the transfer buffer (*see* Fig. 3b). Close the transfer cassette and clamp shut.

4. Place the transfer cassettes into the red/black transfer housing by slotting them down with the black face of each cassette matching the black side of the transfer housing (*see* Fig. 3c).

5. Put the cooling ice pack in the tank next to the side of the transfer housing.

6. Take the 1× transfer buffer from the Pyrex dish and fill the tank—add more as necessary to fill the tank completely to the top covering the transfer housing.

7. Place the tank in the Pyrex dish, put on the cover, and matching red and black cables to probes, attach to the power supply.

8. Turn on the power supply set for 100 V constant and transfer for 1 h.

9. After the run, remove transfer cassettes and open sandwich. Peel back the nitrocellulose from the face of the gel and cut a small notch at in the upper right-hand corner of the nitrocellulose to orient the forward face of the membrane and the top of the gel. The face of the membrane and top will always be oriented with the notch on the upper right. The color markers should serve as a visual metric for the quality of the separation and protein transfer to the membrane.

10. Place the membrane in 1×TBST in a square petri dish on a rocking plate.

3.3 Immuno-detection

1. Wash the membrane 3× for 5 min in 1× TBST in a square petri dish with rocking.

2. Dissolve 10 % nonfat dry milk (NFDM) in TBST with stirring.

3. Cover blot in 10 % NFDM and incubate with rocking for >30 min at room temperature.

4. Wash the membrane 3× for 5 min in 1× TBST in square petri dish with rocking.

5. Using a flat forceps, transfer the membrane to a fresh petri dish or heat-sealed bag, add primary antibody, and incubate ≥3 h at room temperature with rocking. Alternately, overnight incubation at 4 °C can be used. The optimal concentration of a primary antibody should be empirically determined by dilution series.

6. Wash the membrane 3× for 5 min in 1× TBST in a square petri dish with rocking.

7. In a fresh petri dish, add secondary HRP-conjugated antibody and incubate >1 h + at room temperature with rocking. We typically use a secondary antibody at a concentration of 1 μg/mL, but this can be optimized empirically by dilution series.

8. Wash the membrane 3× for 5 min in 1× TBST in a square petri dish with rocking.

9. Prepare enough picoECL SuperSignal substrate by mixing A and B solutions 1:1 just before use to cover the membrane. Be careful not to cross-contaminate the A and B stock solutions.

10. Incubate the membrane in ECL substrate for 5 min with rocking.

11. Place the membrane between a clear sheet of polycarbonate plastic (clear sheet protector), and with a black marker, tick the location of each protein in the ladder using two ticks for the red-colored proteins.

12. Move to imaging device, adjust imager to focus on membrane edge, close door to darken chamber, and collect images at 10 s, 30 s, 1 min, 2 min, and 5 min. Save as TIFF files and annotate the best image with details of the samples and immunoblotting conditions, and print a hard copy as shown in Fig. 4.

4 Notes

1. Optimal sample preparation strategies will vary greatly dependent on the biological source (e.g., plant, yeast, animal), cellular compartment (e.g., nuclear, mitochondrial, cytosolic), and biochemical attributes (e.g., glycosylation, transmembrane) of the protein.

2. Ensure that the method used for quantifying protein is compatible with the extraction buffer. For instance, the Bradford is relatively intolerant to detergent.

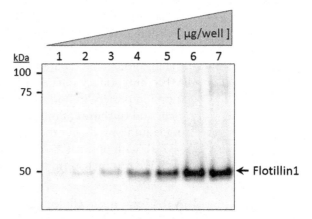

Fig. 4 Western blot for flotillin-1. Increasing amounts of protein (1–7 μg/well) were loaded onto a 4–12 % Bis-Tris gel in MOPS buffer; gel was transferred to nitrocellulose membrane and blotted for the detection of flotillin-1 using a goat-anti-flotillin-1 antibody (1 μg/mL; Santa Cruz Biotech) followed by an HRP-conjugated rabbit anti-mouse secondary antibody (1 μg/m; Jackson ImmunoResearch Labs) with signal resolution using picoECL substrate (Pierce) after 1 min and image recorded using an Alpha Innotech gel documentation system

3. Some antibodies only recognize conformational structures of proteins, epitopes dependent on their 3D shape. These antibodies would be ineffective in the detection of the target antigen following denaturation. Antibodies that tend to recognize a linear or continuous epitope will in general be a better choice for use in detecting denatured proteins by Western blot, and their binding may actually improve upon protein unfolding by exposing epitopes.

4. The intra- and inter-chain disulfide bonds can create complex structural motifs that are insensitive to denaturation. Depending on the location of these chemical bonds to the antibody epitope, their disruption can alter antibody binding.

5. Fluorescent-conjugated primary or secondary antibodies are more appropriate for quantification by Western blot because amplification of signal is linear. Caution should be used when quantifying proteins by Western blot using nonlinear enzyme-linked primary or secondary antibodies.

6. Precast gels offer a convenient cost-effective option to casting your own gels. They come in a variety of formats, thickness, number of wells, and gel percentage with a 16-month shelf life at 4 °C. Generally, we prefer a neutral-pH NuPAGE mini 10 × 10 cm 4–12 % Bis-Tris gradient gel in a 10-well × 1.5 mm thick format that offers the separation of a wide range of molecular weight proteins. The buffering system used is Bis-Tris–HCl (pH 6.4), and MES SDS or MOPS SDS can be used to achieve different

separation ranges of 2–200 and 14–200 kDa, respectively. Gel buffer ions are Bis-Tris$^+$ and Cl$^-$ (pH 6.4) with chloride from the gel buffer serving as the lead ion. MES or MOPS (–) is the trailing ion in the running buffer containing Tris$^+$, MOPS$^-$ or MES$^-$, and dodecylsulfate- (pH 7.3–7.7). Bis-Tris (+) is the common ion present in both gel and running buffer. The number of wells and thickness of the gel will determine the maximum loading volume/well—for the 10-well × 1.5 mm thick mini gel, this is ~37 μL with optimal resolution achieved using ~0.5 μg protein/well. We routinely push this protein load much higher with satisfactory results.

7. A 0.45 μm nitrocellulose filter paper is recommended for most Western blotting applications and we prefer the precut and preassembled blotting membrane filter paper sets. Nonsupported nitrocellulose is brittle and care should be taken when handling. PVDF membranes are an equally viable alternative to nitrocellulose; they are more expensive but provide strong protein transfer, reduced nonspecific protein binding during Western blotting, and compatibility with downstream mass spectrometry applications. PVDF requires methanol for wetting.

8. Equal volume load is important to ensure an even run of the sample through the gel. Adjust volumes as necessary using a 1× LDS buffer and do not leave the well empty; always add 1 × LDS buffer blank to avoid band spreading.

9. You should see fine bubbles in the tank if the current is flowing. MES buffer runs faster than MOPS. Use the bromophenol blue dye front and the colorimetric protein ladder to evaluate protein separation and run time. If you run the gel too long, you will run the protein off the gel.

References

1. Mahmood T, Yang PC (2012) Western blot: technique, theory, and trouble shooting. N Am J Med Sci 4:429–434

2. Weiss W, Görg A (2008) Sample solubilization buffers for two-dimensional electrophoresis. Methods Mol Biol 424:35–42

3. Cordwell SJ (2008) Sequential extraction of proteins by chemical reagents. Methods Mol Biol 424:139–146

4. Friedenauer S, Berlet HH (1989) Sensitivity and variability of the Bradford protein assay in the presence of detergents. Anal Biochem 178:263–268

5. Walker JM (1994) The bicinchoninic acid (BCA) assay for protein quantitation. Methods Mol Biol 32:5–8

6. Kurien BT, Scofield RH (2006) Western blotting. Methods 38:283–293

7. Fowler SJ (1995) Use of monoclonal antibodies for western blotting with enhanced chemiluminescent detection. Methods Mol Biol 45:115–127

8. Alegria-Schaffer A, Lodge A, Vattem K (2009) Performing and optimizing Western blots with an emphasis on chemiluminescent detection. Methods Enzymol 463:573–599

9. Sandhu GS, Eckloff BW, Kline BC (1991) Chemiluminescent substrates increase sensitivity of antigen detection in western blots. Biotechniques 11:14–16

10. Dubitsky A, DeCollibus D, Ortolano GA (2002) Sensitive fluorescent detection of protein on nylon membranes. J Biochem Biophys Methods 51:47–56

11. MacPhee DJ (2010) Methodological considerations for improving Western blot analysis. J Pharmacol Toxicol Methods 61:171–177

Chapter 10

Flow-Through Assay for Detection of Antibodies Using Protein-A Colloidal Gold Conjugate as a Probe

Sreedevi Chennuru and Panduranga Rao Pavuluri

Abstract

Flow-through assay (FTA) is a rapid, simple-to-perform, cost-effective, and user-friendly diagnostic test for monitoring infections in non-laboratory settings. It is mostly applied for antibody detection. FTA employing protein-A colloidal gold conjugate to detect antibodies against porcine cysticerci using cyst fluid and whole cyst antigens of *Taenia solium* metacestode is described here. Antibodies in the serum are captured by an antigen spotted onto a nitrocellulose membrane mounted on a flow-through device that serves as the antigen capture matrix. The bound antibodies are visualized by the addition of protein-A colloidal gold conjugate, which imparts a pink color. The test can be completed within 3 min at room temperature without any instrumentation. The sensitivity and specificity of the FTA are in agreement with ELISA.

Key words Flow-through assay, Nitrocellulose membrane, Antibodies, Colloidal gold conjugate

1 Introduction

Immunodiagnostics play a very important role in disease diagnosis. Initial immunodiagnostics were based on the radiolabeling of an antigen or antibody and were limited to a few sophisticated well-equipped labs. With the advent of the enzyme-linked immunosorbent assay (ELISA) and other non-radiolabeled immunoassays, the use of immunodiagnostics became more popular. The major limitations of ELISA are (a) its microplate format which is more suitable for surveillance or for big hospital settings rather than for individual samples, and when inordinate, waiting time may be imposed till enough samples have accumulated, (b) time and trained manpower required for testing, and (c) specialized equipment to determine cutoffs for positive and negative samples. Three different immunoassays are being used for the diagnosis of infectious agents based on membrane matrices, i.e., lateral flow assay (LFA), dot immunobinding assay (DIA) or flow-through assay (FTA), and dipstick assay (DSA). These tests are often referred to as rapid diagnostic tests (RDTs), bedside tests, pen-

Robert Hnasko (ed.), *ELISA: Methods and Protocols*, Methods in Molecular Biology, vol. 1318,
DOI 10.1007/978-1-4939-2742-5_10, © Springer Science+Business Media New York 2015

side tests, or point-of-care tests (POCT). Most of the RDTs are semiquantitative or qualitative tests, simply differentiating between positive and negative by the development of a dot or change in color or development of a colored line. These systems are useful in resource-limited laboratories and hospitals and also to take quick decisions on the course of treatment without waiting for the results of time-consuming tests like ELISA or immunoblotting. In all three assays, the principle is the same, i.e., antigen-antibody complex formation and visualization of the complex through color developed from a chromogenic substrate. All these qualitative assays are also less time consuming and can be employed without any need of equipment and training.

Flow-through assay is a rapid test as the total procedure is completed within 3–5 min, is simple to perform, is cost-effective, and can be performed with minimal training without any laboratory equipment. Several studies have reported the use of FTA for the detection of hormones, insecticides, viral antigens, and serum antibodies [1–3]. Though these tests can be used to detect both antibodies and antigens, sensitivity is more for antibody detection assays [3–5], although the detection of antigen is often less sensitive than lateral flow or traditional enzyme immunoassay (EIA) methods [2]. However, FTAs are preferred over lateral flow tests for the simultaneous diagnosis of multiple concurrently occurring pathogens, e.g., multiple rapid HIV/HCV (MedMira) antibody test [6].

Before developing any FTA system, one needs to decide the analyte to be detected, i.e., antigen or antibodies (*see* **Note 1**). Among the reagents to be used, one needs to consider the following points before planning for the development of the assay: (a) type of antigens, i.e., proteins (native or recombinant), peptides, and polysaccharides, as well as the purity of the antigen; (b) type of antibodies (monoclonal or polyclonal) and their specificity, affinity, and avidity; (c) the most suitable format for detection, i.e., direct, indirect, competition, inhibition, etc.; and (d) chromogenic substance. Unlike enzyme-based color development, colloidal dye particles are used in FTA (*see* **Note 2**). Initially, colloidal gold-conjugated antibody or antigen for the detection of antigen or antibody, respectively, was used on a nitrocellulose membrane in dot immunobinding assay [7–10]. Subsequently, colloidal gold-labeled protein A is being used as a probe for the detection of antibodies in serum samples [3–5, 11]. For immunoblotting, membrane-based matrices are used along with an absorbent material (*see* **Note 3**).

The development of an FTA for detection of antibodies to parasites belonging to *Taenia solium* is described here employing porcine cysticercosis as a model. Antigens in the form of cyst fluid (CF) and whole cyst (WC) antigens of *Taenia solium* metacestodes coated onto nitrocellulose membrane and test sera are probed with a protein-A colloidal gold conjugate. The sensitivity and specificity of FTA were in agreement with those of ELISA when conducted with CF and WC antigens [3]. The whole procedure could be completed in 3–5 min at room temperature with visualized results of colored spots.

2 Materials

1. Flow-through modules contain an absorbing pad between upper and lower plastic casings (*see* Fig. 1) (*see* **Note 3**).

2. Nitrocellulose membrane, 0.45 μm pore size (*see* **Note 3**).

3. Wash solution [phosphate-buffered saline—Tween 20 (PBST), pH 7.4]: 0.20 g potassium chloride, 0.20 g potassium dihydrogen orthophosphate, 8.00 g sodium chloride, and 1.16 g disodium hydrogen phosphate are dissolved in 800 ml of distilled water, 5 ml of Tween 20 is added, and the solution is made up to 1,000 ml.

4. Blocking solution: dissolve 5 g of skimmed milk powder (any high-quality powder available in grocery store) in 100 ml of PBST (*see* **Note 4**).

5. Antigens: cyst fluid antigen (CFA) and whole cyst antigen (WCA). Prepare CFA and WCA as reported [12, 13] (*see* **Note 5**).

6. Conjugates: colloidal gold conjugate (*see* **Note 2**).

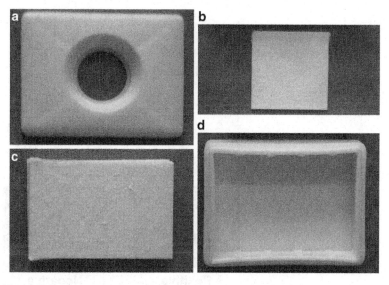

Fig. 1 Flow-though device: (**a**) Upper casing, (**b**) nitrocellulose membrane, (**c**) absorbent pad, (**d**) lower casing

3   Methods

Flow-through assay (FTA) for antibody detection (*see* Fig. 2): The procedure can be divided into two components, i.e., antigen coating and testing sera for antibodies. The procedure described here includes the preparation of antigen-coated devices for future use. However, the procedure can be modified to prepare a few devices and use them immediately (*see* ref. [3]). Carry out all procedures at room temperature unless specified otherwise.

Test principle: In the assay, antibodies in the serum sample are captured by an antigen spotted onto a nitrocellulose membrane mounted on a flow-through device that serves as the antigen

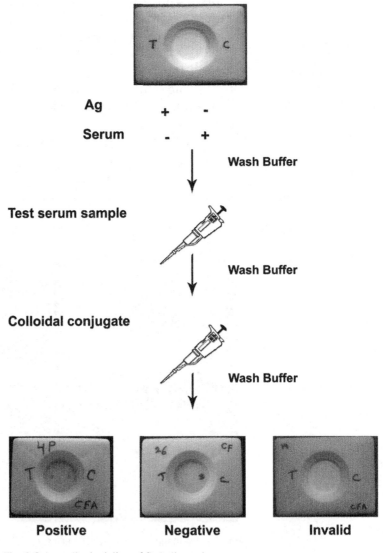

Fig. 2 Schematic depiction of flow-through assay

capture matrix. The bound antibodies are visualized by the addition of protein-A colloidal gold conjugate, which imparts a pink color to the membrane.

3.1 Antigen Coating

1. Place the nitrocellulose membrane on a blotting paper (*see* **Note 6**).

2. Place 1 μl (250 ng/μl) of antigen at one end ("T" side) and 1 μl of pig serum at the opposite end ("C" side) (*see* **Note 7**).

3. Dry the membrane in an incubator at 37 °C for 1 h or at room temperature overnight (*see* **Note 8**).

4. Wash the membrane with 200 μl of wash buffer and allow wicking through the membrane by capillary action (*see* **Note 9**).

5. Dip the membranes in blocking buffer, incubate at 4 °C for 1 h, place the membrane on blotting paper, and dry the membrane by incubating at 37 °C for 1 h or at room temperature overnight (*see* **Note 10**).

6. Place the membrane in flow-through module making sure that the membrane is tightly in contact with the underlying absorbing pad (*see* **Note 6**).

3.2 Testing Sera for Antibodies

1. Add 200 μl of test serum diluted 1:10 in wash buffer and allow it to be absorbed through the membrane (*see* **Note 11**).

2. Add 200 μl of wash buffer and wait until the buffer is absorbed completely.

3. Add 200 μl of protein-A colloidal gold conjugate diluted 1:2 in wash buffer and allow to be absorbed through the membrane (*see* **Note 12**).

4. Add 200 μl of wash buffer and wait until the buffer is absorbed completely.

5. Appearances of two pink dots indicate the presence of antibodies and indicate that the test is positive. Appearance of no color at T dot with pink color at C dot indicates that the result is negative. If no pink color appears at C dot, the test is invalid and the test needs to be repeated (*see* **Note 7**).

4 Notes

1. Immunodiagnostics can be basically divided in to two systems, i.e., those that detect the antigen or the etiological agent and those that detect antibodies against the agent. These tests respectively employ specific antibodies or antigens. Antigen detection is more useful for acute diseases (e.g., dengue fever, malaria) and to detect an ongoing infection and can assist

clinicians to tailor treatment regimen. This includes the detection of whole organism or parts of it. The identification of antibodies from the patient's serum is more useful for the diagnosis of chronic infections like those caused by hepatitis B and human immunodeficiency viruses. The use of antibody detection assays cannot differentiate the current versus previous infections unless antibody types are detected, e.g., identification of IgM antibodies for the detection of ongoing dengue infection. As a corollary, such tests will be misleading in endemic areas because most of the population shows detectable level of antibodies owing to prior exposure to the specific or a closely related pathogen. For instance, both ELISA and RDT tests for tuberculosis are discouraged for use in endemic areas (*see* ref. [14]). On the other hand, antibody detection tests are more useful for epidemiological surveys and are the only assays used for the detection of vaccine-induced antibodies.

2. In ELISA and EIA, an enzyme is conjugated to the antigen or antibody and the detection is based on the production of color when the substrate is converted to a colored substance by the enzyme. In rapid assays, colloidal gold is conjugated to antibodies or protein A, G, or A/G (though colloidal nonmetals like selenium are available, gold conjugates are more popular; colloidal conjugated protein A and antibodies are commercially available). Proteins A, G, and L are naturally occurring immunoglobulin-binding proteins produced by bacteria. Proteins A and G bind to the Fc portion of antibodies, whereas protein L binds to the light chain of antibodies in the Fab region. All these proteins differ in their antibody-binding specificities and a recombinant protein A/G has broader antibody specificity than either of proteins A or G. The selection of protein A, G, or A/G also depends on the antibody type and species. Since proteins A and G do not or weakly bind IgM, the detection of IgM antibodies is best achieved using anti-IgM antibodies conjugated with colloidal gold. Hence, it is essential to carry out a pilot assay to test the binding of the conjugated protein A/G to the antibodies being used. If a sandwich test is used, where an antigen is sandwiched between two types of antibodies, anti-immunoglobulin conjugates are more preferable than protein A/G conjugates. Different sizes of colloidal gold particles are available for different applications. In general, for immunoblotting assays, colloidal gold particles of >15 nm size are used (20 nm size particles are commercially available).

3. Different matrices are available for coating the proteins. Nitrocellulose membranes are considered most suitable for FTAs. Pore size of the membrane plays an important role in

coating and assay time. Pore sizes from 0.22 to 0.45 μm are generally used. Higher pore sizes are used for other assays like LFA. Protein binding is better with membranes with smaller pore size. In addition, the flow rate is slower allowing enough time for the antibody to bind. Together, higher protein binding and slow flow rate produce higher sensitivity. On the other hand, slow flow rate can also lead to higher background and longer assay times. Different absorbent materials are available for fluid absorption, and the thickness of the absorbent pad and its absorption capacity need to be considered based on the volume of the fluid (sample, wash buffer) or the number of washes being used in the test. In general, pads that can absorb 4 ml of liquid are suitable for FTA. Care should be exercised to keep the absorbent pad in close contact with the membrane for proper flow of the reagents during the assay; hence, the thickness of the pad should be sufficient to keep the pad and membrane in close apposition.

4. In FTA, antigens/antibodies are applied to the nitrocellulose membranes as small dots, and binding of the proteins to the membrane is based on non-covalent interactions. Drying of proteins on the membrane results in the binding of the proteins to the membrane. As the assays do not involve prolonged incubation, nonspecific binding of antibodies to the membrane is rarely observed, and hence, most of the manufacturers suggest using the membranes without blocking. In case of high nonspecific background, blocking agents can be used. In general, membranes are dipped in concentrated (1–5 %) protein solutions to block uncoated areas of the membranes. Common proteins used are bovine serum albumin (BSA), skimmed milk powder (nonfat dry milk), and fish gelatin in PBS. It is not advised to use sera for blocking as antibodies present in the sera will produce nonspecific reactivity on the whole membrane.

5. The adsorption of proteins to the membrane is based on non-covalent interactions and the antigens or antibodies need to be prepared in coating buffer. The pH of the coating buffer plays an important role in the adsorption to the nitrocellulose membrane. Availability of pKa values of the proteins to be adsorbed will be helpful in deciding the pH of the coating buffer, i.e., the pH of the buffer should be more than the pKa value of the proteins. In general, buffer pH values between 8 and 9 work well with most of the proteins. The source of the proteins also plays an important role.

6. The antigen-coated membranes can either be used immediately or stored and used later. Antigen coating is the most time-consuming step in the assembly of the flow-through devices. In general, kits are prepared in bulk and stored for future use. For one-time usage, instead of using blotting paper,

the membrane can be placed directly over the absorbing pad in the FTA module (*see* ref. [3]).

7. The serum will be coated on the control (C) side of the strip. This will act as control for protein-A colloidal gold conjugate binding to antibodies. Colloidal gold-conjugated protein A will bind to this dot and a pink color is produced. The C dot should turn to pink once colloidal gold-conjugated protein A is added to the test device. No color development at the C dot is an indication of test failure and the test needs to be repeated. Test antigen (T) will be placed on the other side of the strip. Care should be taken to place the C and T dots at least 0.5 cm apart. Specific antibodies binding to the antigen are then bound by a colloidal gold conjugate, developing into a pink dot in case of positive test, and no color development is considered negative for specific antibodies.

8. If an incubator is not available for drying the flow-through modules, drying can be achieved by overnight incubation at room temperature. Care should be exercised to dry the membrane completely. The proteins bind to the membrane by non-covalent interactions and stability of the bound proteins will be more when the membrane is completely dried.

9. Washing of the membrane will remove the unbound antigen.

10. This step can be avoided when background is not a problem (*see* **Note 4**).

11. The dilution of sera to be used is dictated by the quantity of the serum available to test. An initial dilution of 1:5 is suggested. However, if background is an issue, higher dilutions can then be tested. During our preliminary experiments, 1 in 100 serum dilutions provided clear pink-colored dots, but lightly infected pig (on meat inspection) serum samples gave very faint dots. Hence, further dilutions were made and finally 1 in 10 dilutions was found to be optimum even for light infections and it makes the test reagent conservative (*see* ref. [4, 15]).

12. Most of the manufacturers supply colloidal gold conjugates in concentrated form and working concentration of conjugate needs to be determined empirically. Dilutions ranging from two to tenfold should be tested for each batch of the colloidal gold conjugate being used.

Acknowledgments

The authors sincerely acknowledge Dr. Nagendra R. Hegde for the critical review of the manuscript.

References

1. Wang S, Zhang C, Zhang Y (2005) Development of a flow-through enzyme linked immunosorbent assay and a dipstick assay for the rapid detection of insecticide caraxyl. Acta Chim Acta 535:219–225

2. Subramanyam KV, Purushothaman V, Muralimanohar B et al (2012) Development of Single Serum ELISA and Flow Through Assay for Infectious Bursal Disease of Poultry. J Adv Vet Res 2:113–119

3. Sreedevi C, Md H, Subramanyam KV et al (2011) Development and evaluation of flow through assay for detection of antibodies against porcine cysticercosis. Trop Biomed 28:160–170

4. Dubinsky P, Akao N, Reiterova K et al (2000) Comparison of the sensitive screening kit with two ELISA sets for detection of anti-toxocara antibodies. Southeast Asian J Trop Med Public Health 31:394–398

5. Gan XX, Yue W, Xun GJ et al (2006) Development of dot immunogold filtration assay kit for rapid detection of specific antibodies against Cysticercus cellulosae. J Trop Med 1:17–19

6. Smith BD, Drobeniuc J, Jewett A et al (2011) Evaluation of three rapid screening assays for detection of antibodies to hepatitis C virus. J Infect Dis 204:825–831

7. Kashiwazaki Y, Snowden K, Smith DH et al (1994) A multiple antigen detection dipstick colloidal dye immunoassay for the field diagnosis of trypanosome infection in cattle. Vet Parasitol 55:57–69

8. Mistrello G, Gentili M, Falagini P et al (1995) Dot immunobinding assay as a new diagnostic test for human hydatid disease. Immunol Lett 47:79–95

9. Xiao X, Wang T, Tian Z (2003) Development of rapid, sensitive, dye immunoassay for schistosomosis diagnosis: a colloidal dye immunofiltration assay. J Immunol Methods 280:49–57

10. Ali IO, Sibel E, Salih E et al (2005) Diagnostic Value of a dot immunobinding assay for human pulmonary hydatidosis. Korean J Parasitol 43:15–18

11. Eliades P, Karagouni E, Stergiatou I et al (1998) A simple method for the serodiagnosis of human hydatid disease based on a protein A/colloidal dye conjugate. J Immunol Methods 218:123–132

12. Chung JY, Eom KS, Yang Y et al (2005) A seroepidemiological survey of Taenia solium cysticercosis in Nabo, Guangxi Zhuang Autonomous Region, China. Korean J Parasitol 43:135–139

13. Mahajan RC, Chiktara NL, Chopra JS (1974) Evaluation of cysticercus and adult worm antigens in serodiagnosis of cysticercosis. Indian J Med Res 62:1310–1313

14. Steingart KR, Ramsay A, Dowdy DW et al (2012) Serological tests for the diagnosis of active tuberculosis: relevance for India. Indian J Med Res 135:695–702

15. Wan OA, Sulaiman O, Yusof S et al (2001) Epidemiological screening of lymphatic filariasis among immigrants using dipstick colloidal dye immuno assay. Malays J Med Sci 8:19–24

Chapter 11

Multiplexed Microsphere Suspension Array-Based Immunoassays

Andrew Lin, Alexandra Salvador, and J. Mark Carter

Abstract

ELISA is an extremely powerful tool to detect analytes because of its sensitivity, selectivity, reproducibility and ease of use. Here we describe sandwich immunoassays performed in suspension on spectrally unique microspheres developed by Luminex. Luminex assays offer the benefit of multiplex analysis of large numbers of analytes in a single reaction. Because the microspheres are spectrally unique, many microspheres, each attached to various antibodies, can be added to a single sample. Luminex instruments can distinguish each microsphere and detect the intensity of a reporter signal for each microsphere. Results are reported in Median Fluorescent Intensities for each analyte. Luminex assays can be used to detect up to 500 analytes in a high-throughput format. Luminex refers to this technology as xMAP®. Here we describe a routine protocol for a Luminex immunoassay. Other Luminex assays would have to be optimized for specific conditions according to their use.

Key words Microsphere, Bead-based assay, ELISA, Immunoassay, Antibody, Multiplex

1 Introduction

While immunoassays have been driving advances in such areas as life science research, clinical diagnostics, biosurveillance, and food safety, recent developments in microsphere-based immunoassay technology may provide further improvements. With microsphere suspension-based arrays, it is possible to perform multiplex analyses, simultaneous analysis of multiple analytes in a single reaction, which can generate more data with less sample, reduced labor, cost, and analysis time. With traditional microplate ELISA, it is possible to perform high-throughput analysis, but only multiplex 5–10 different analytes at a time [1]. By contrast protein microarrays can multiplex hundreds of analyses but with limited throughput and accuracy [2]. With microsphere-based suspension arrays, it is possible to multiplex up to 500 analyses in a high-throughput format.

Robert Hnasko (ed.), *ELISA: Methods and Protocols*, Methods in Molecular Biology, vol. 1318, DOI 10.1007/978-1-4939-2742-5_11, © Springer Science+Business Media New York 2015

Luminex xMAP technology uses microspheres of a single size (5.6 μm) but with unique ratios of infrared and red internal dyes. Each microsphere set, therefore, fluoresces with a unique spectral ratio of these two wavelengths when the internal dyes are excited. The microspheres are available with a carboxylic acid modification of their surface. These can be covalently coupled to antibodies for analyte capture on the microsphere's surface. Subsequent detection is via a biotinylated detector antibody in a sandwich immunoassay format (*see* **Note 1**). After the addition of a fluorescent reporter (i.e., typically streptavidin–phycoerythrin), Luminex instruments can be used to analyze each sandwich immunoassay. Because each microsphere set features a unique spectral address, multiple assays (i.e., on microspheres attached to different antibodies) can be combined in a single reaction (*see* Fig. 1). Luminex instruments separate the microspheres for individual analysis by lining them up in a one-dimensional array via flow cytometry (i.e., Luminex 100, 200, and FlexMAP 3D), or by spreading them in a two-dimensional monolayer (i.e., MagPix). The 1D arrays are read, one bead at a time, via interrogation with a set of red and green lasers, while the 2D arrays are read via hyperspectral imaging using LED excitation and CCD imagery. The multiplex format of

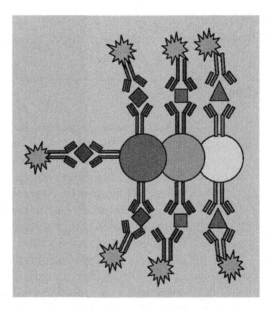

Fig. 1 Schematic showing different bead sets with different spectral characteristics, each coupled to a different capture Ab, recognizing its respective different antigen. Detection is accomplished by using a single streptavidin probe that reacts with all biotinylated capture antibodies. In this diagram the color of the Ab implies that the same Ab is used for both capture and detection. Sometimes this works, especially for polyclonal Ab, although best results are obtained with the use of monoclonal Ab, with a different specificity in the capture and detection Ab

Luminex microsphere-based immunoassays allows for the detection of up to 50 analytes on the MagPix platform, 100 analytes on the Luminex 100 and 200, or 500 analytes on the FlexMap 3D in high throughput 96- or 384-well formats (*see* **Note 2**).

All of these instruments determine which analyte is being measured through one fluorescent channel (i.e., the red microsphere internal dye), and the intensity of the signal through a second fluorescent channel (i.e., the green phycoerythrin tag), providing a readout in median fluorescent intensity (MFI) for each target (*see* **Note 3**). With the large surface area to volume ratio of the 5.6 μm microspheres, up to 100,000 capture antibody molecules can be coupled per microsphere. This relatively high density facilitates antigen binding for excellent sensitivity. Furthermore, because of the small size of the microspheres, the kinetics of the binding reactions approach solution-phase kinetics, even while the solid-phase nature of the microspheres forces the binding reaction equilibrium to favor the bound state. As with microplate format immunoassays, quantitative analysis may be performed using external standards to generate standard curves. Multiplex capability also facilitates the use of internal standards to correct for variations due to sample processing.

Luminex type immunoassays provide at least two major advantages over traditional antibody microarrays. One is that a user may choose to run any subset of the multiplex, conserving assay reagents and analysis time, while a microarray requires use of the entire array. Even more significantly, to be practical and economical, microarrays are printed at a commercial scale, and the user must choose between and among commercial offerings. On the other hand, the Luminex format allows a user to create individual assays and combine them to make custom multiplex assays. That particular benefit is the primary subject of this discussion. Furthermore, when MagPlex beads are used, a third significant advantage becomes apparent, because in this case the sandwich ELISA comprises an immunomagnetic pull-down experiment. A few thousand microspheres may effectively interrogate up to 50 mL of sample, recovering the analyte for further characterization [3].

2   Materials

Coupling Capture Antibody to MagPlex-C Magnetic Carboxylated Microspheres

1. Capture antibodies.

2. MagPlex Microspheres (Luminex Corporation, Austin, TX) (*see* **Note 4**). One microsphere region for each target analyte. Refer to manufacturer's recommendation for compatible microsphere regions for multiplex assays.

3. LoBind Eppendorf microcentrifuge tube (Eppendorf, Hauppauge, NY).

4. Activation Buffer: 0.1 M NaH_2PO_4, pH 6.2. Weigh 3 g Sodium phosphate monobasic, anhydrous (Sigma-Aldrich, St. Louis, MO) bring to 200 mL with dI water. Mix and adjust pH to 6.2 with 5 N NaOH (Fisher Scientific, Pittsburgh, PA) (*see* **Note 5**). Bring to 250 mL. Filter-sterilize and store at 4 °C, up to several weeks.

5. PBS pH 7.4. 0.01 M phosphate buffered saline with 138 mM NaCl, 2.7 mM KCl (Sigma-Aldrich). Weigh one packet of powder PBS. Bring up to 1 L with water. Filter-sterilize and store at 4 °C, up to several weeks (*see* **Note 6**).

6. S-NHS: N-hydroxysulfosuccinimide (Thermo Scientific Pierce Protein Biology Products, Rockford, IL) Store at–20 °C. Warm to room temperature in a desiccator 1 h prior to use. Make fresh 50 mg/mL S-NHS in Activation Buffer on day of use.

7. EDC: 1-ethyl-3-(3-dimethylaminopropyl) carbodiimide (Thermo Scientific Pierce Protein Biology Products). Store at–20 °C. Warm to room temperature in desiccator 1 h prior to use. Make fresh 50 mg/mL EDC in Activation Buffer immediately before use.

8. PBS–TBN: 0.01 M phosphate buffered saline with 137 mM NaCl 2.7 mM KCl, 0.1 % BSA, 0.02 % Tween 20, 0.05 % sodium azide, pH 7.4. To one packet of PBS (Sigma-Aldrich), add 1 g of BSA (Sigma-Aldrich), 0.2 mL of Tween 20 (Sigma-Aldrich), and 500 mg of sodium azide (Sigma, Aldrich). Bring up to 1 L with water. Filter-sterilize and store at 4 °C, for up to 1 year.

9. Equipment needed: vortex mixer, Branson 200 Ultrasonic Cleaner (Branson Ultrasonics Corp. Danbury, CT) or equivalent sonicating water bath, Dynal RotaMix Rotator (Life Technologies, Grand Island, NY) or equivalent rotator, DynaMag-2 Magnetic Particle Concentrator (Life Technologies) or equivalent magnetic separator for 1.5 mL microcentrifuge tubes, hemacytometer, light microscope.

Confirmation of Capture Antibody Coupling

1. PBS–1 % BSA: 0.01 M Phosphate Buffered Saline with 137 mM NaCl 2.7 mM KCl, 0.1 % BSA, pH 7.4. To one packet of PBS add 10 g BSA (Sigma-Aldrich). Bring up to 1 L with water. Filter-sterilize and store at 4 °C, up to 4 weeks.

2. PE-antispecies IgG: R-Phycoerythrin-labeled anti-species IgG antibodies (Life Technologies). Use appropriate PE-antispecies IgG to species of capture antibody. Dilute in PBS–1 % BSA to appropriate dilution.

3. Equipment: Black 96-well round bottom polystyrene microtiter plate (Corning Costar, Lowell, MA), LifeSep 96 F Magnetic Separator (Dexter Magnetic Technologies, Elk Grove Village, IL)

or equivalent 96-well plate magnetic separator, IKA MTS 2/4 Digital (IKA Works, Inc., Wilmington, NC) or equivalent plate shaker, Luminex 100, 200, FlexMap 3D or MagPix (Luminex Corp.) or any Luminex technology supported platform.

Immunoassay

1. PBS–1 % BSA

2. Capture Ab-Magplex: Capture antibody conjugated to Magplex microspheres as described below, diluted into PBS–1 % BSA.

3. Biotinylated Detector Ab: Detector antibody conjugated to biotin, diluted in PBS–1 % BSA (*see* **Note 7**).

4. SAPE: Streptavidin–R-Phycoerythrin (Life Technologies). Dilute SAPE to 4 µg/mL in PBS–1 % BSA.

5. Equipment: IKA MTS 2/4 digital plate shaker, vortex, LifeSep 96 F magnetic separator

Luminex 100/200

1. Sheath Fluid (Bio-Rad Laboratories, Hercules, CA).

2. 70 % isopropanol.

3. Bleach.

4. DI water.

5. Bio-Plex Calibration Kit (Bio-Rad Laboratories).

6. Bio-Plex Validation Kit 4.0 (Bio-Rad Laboratories).

MAGPIX

1. MAGPIX Calibration Kit (Luminex Corp.).

2. MAGPIX Performance Verification Kit (Luminex Corp.).

3. 70 % isopropanol.

4. 0.1 N NaOH.

3 Methods

3.1 Coupling Capture Antibody to Microspheres

For each target, couple capture antibody to spectrally unique microsphere. For multiplex reactions, ensure that microsphere regions are compatible by referring to manufacturer's recommendations (*see* **Note 8**). Microspheres and SAPE should be protected from prolonged exposure to light (*see* **Note 9**).

1. Resuspend MagPlex microspheres by gently rotating at 20 rpm, 1–2 min for 1 mL of microspheres, or 10–15 min for 4 mL of microspheres.

2. Transfer 5×10^6 microspheres to LoBind Eppendorf tubes. Place tube in DynaMag-2 Magnetic Particle Concentrator for 30–60 s and use a micropipette to carefully remove supernatant from the small pellet.

3. Remove tube from magnetic separator for 30–60 s and resuspend microspheres in 100 µL dH$_2$O. Vortex for 20 s, and sonicate for additional 20 s to obtain a homogenous suspension.

4. Place tube in magnetic separator for 30–60 s and remove supernatant. Resuspend microspheres in 80 µL Activation Buffer. Vortex for 20 s and sonicate for additional 20 s.

5. Add 10 µL S-NHS 50 mg/mL to microspheres. Mix by vortexing.

6. Add 10 µL EDC 50 mg/mL. Mix by vortexing.

7. Cover coupling reaction tubes with aluminum foil and rotate at room temperature for 20 min.

8. Place tube in magnetic separator for 30–60 s and remove supernatant.

9. Remove tube from magnetic separator and resuspend microspheres in 150 µL of PBS pH 7.4. Mix by vortexing. Pellet using magnet, and remove and discard supernatant. Repeat wash in 150 µL PBS, then resuspend in 100 µL PBS.

10. Add 5–12 µg of capture antibody. Adjust final volume to 500 µL with PBS. Cover reaction tube in aluminum foil and rotate at room temperature for 2 h. Alternatively, agitate microspheres on rotator overnight in darkness at 4 °C.

11. Place tube in magnetic separator 30–60 s and remove supernatant.

12. Resuspend microspheres in 500 µL PBS–TBN. Vortex for 20 s and sonicate for additional 20 s. Cover coupling reaction tubes in aluminum foil and agitate microspheres on rotator at room temperature for 30 min.

13. Place tube in magnetic separator 30–60 s and resuspend microspheres in 1 mL PBS–TBN. Mix by vortexing 20 s and sonicating for 20 s.

14. Place tube in magnetic separator for 30–60 s, remove and discard supernatant, and repeat 1 mL PBS–TBN wash.

15. Resuspend microspheres in 250–1,000 µL PBS–TBN.

16. Determine microsphere concentration with hemacytometer on the microscope, according to the manufacturer's instructions. Store coupled microspheres at 4 °C protected from light, for up to 1 year.

3.2 Confirmation of Capture Antibody Coupling

1. Resuspend microspheres by vortexing for 20 s and sonicating for 20 s.

2. Prepare working microsphere mixture by diluting microspheres to 100 microspheres/µL in PBS–1 % BSA.

3. Prepare twofold serial dilutions (4–0.5 µg/mL) of phycoerythrin labeled anti-species IgG antibodies using the correct species for each respective capture antibody, diluted in PBS–1 % BSA.

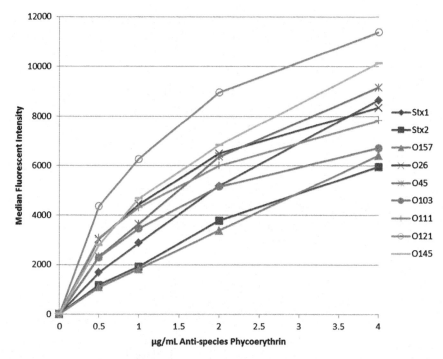

Fig. 2 Confirmation of Capture Antibody Coupling to Microspheres. Capture antibodies to shigatoxin 1, shigatoxin 2, and the lipopolysaccharides various *E. coli* O serogroups (rabbit anti-O45 and O145, mouse anti-stx1, stx2, and O157, goat anti-O26, O103, O111, and O121) were coupled to MagPlex Microspheres [3]. Microspheres were tested using 5,000 beads with 0–4 µg/mL of the corresponding anti-species Phycoerythrin

4. Add 50 µL working microsphere mixture to microtiter plate wells, with additional well for negative control (i.e., no PE-labeled anti-species Ab).

5. Add 50 µL of each PE labeled anti-species detector to each of the appropriate wells. Add 50 µL PBS–1 % BSA to negative control well.

6. Cover microtiter plate in foil and incubate at room temperature for 30 min with agitation on plate shaker.

7. Place microtiter plate on 96-well plate magnetic separator for 30–60 s and remove supernatant.

8. Wash microspheres in 100 µL PBS–1 % BSA twice.

9. Resuspend microspheres in 100 µL PBS–1 % BSA. Mix by pipetting.

10. Analyze on Luminex instrument (*see* Fig. 2).

3.3 Immunoassay

1. Resuspend microspheres by vortexing for 20 s and sonicating for 20 s.

2. Construct a multiplex assay by combining 100 microsphere/µL of each set of microsphere in a single microcentrifuge tube.

Place tube on magnetic separator 30–60 s and remove supernatant. Resuspend in PBS–1 % BSA to a concentration of 100 of each microsphere/μL and mix by vortex for 20 s and sonication for 20 s.

3. Aliquot 50 μL of microsphere mixture to appropriate wells of microtiter plate (enough wells for samples + background) (*see* **Note 10**).

4. Add 50 μL PBS–1 % BSA to background well.

5. Add 50 μL sample to appropriate wells.

6. Mix by pipetting. Cover plate in foil and place on plate shaker at 800 rpm for 30 min at room temperature.

7. Place plate on magnetic separator for 30–60 s and remove supernatant.

8. Wash microspheres 2× in 100 μL PBS–1 % BSA (*see* **Note 11**).

9. Remove plate from magnetic separator and resuspend microspheres in 50 μL PBS–1 % BSA, mixing with a micropipette.

10. Prepare detector antibody mixture by adding all detector antibodies to single tube. Dilute to 1–4 μg/mL each antibody in PBS–1 % BSA. Add 50 μL detector antibody mixture to each well. Mix by pipetting.

11. Cover plate in foil and place on plate shaker at 800 rpm for 30 min at room temperature.

12. Place the plate on magnetic separator for 30–60 s and remove supernatant.

13. Wash microspheres 2× in 100 μL PBS–1 % BSA.

14. Remove plate from magnetic separator and resuspend microspheres in 50 μL PBS–1 % BSA.

15. Dilute Streptavidin–R-Phycroerythrin to 4 μg/mL in PBS–1 % BSA and add 50 μL to each well.

16. Cover plate in foil and place on plate shaker at 800 rpm for 30 min at room temperature.

17. Place the plate on magnetic separator for 30–60 s and remove supernatant.

18. Wash microspheres 2× in 100 μL PBS–1 % BSA.

19. Remove plate from magnetic separator and resuspend microspheres in 100 μL PBS–1 % BSA. Mix by pipetting.

20. Analyze microspheres on Luminex technology supported system.

3.4 Luminex Analysis

Perform daily startup, optics warm-up, calibration, validation, and sample height adjustment according to owner's manual. Ensure that waste container is empty, and sheath fluid is adequately full before use. After each day of use, perform shutdown (*see* **Note 12**).

1. In Bio-Plex Manager v 6.0 (*see* **Note 13**), in describe protocol menu, click add panel. Enter < panel name > and select correct assay < Bio-Plex MagPlex Beads (Magnetic) >.

2. In < Select Analyte > menu, click < Add Panel > button to open the < Add Analyte > window. Enter appropriate Microsphere Region number and name of analyte for that region. Repeat until all multiplexed microsphere regions and targets are entered.

3. In < Select Analyte > window. Highlight desired microsphere region/targets from available list and click add button to move to the selected list (*see* **Note 14**).

4. In Format Plate menu, Plate Formatting Tab, define which wells in 96-well plate to analyze. Click Blank button, then highlight well or wells that contain blank (all components except for analyte). Click unknown button, then highlight appropriate wells with sample. Wells with unknown samples will be numbered.

5. In Format Plate, Plate Groupings tab can be used to define a group to calculate signal to background ratios for each well. Highlight all wells to be grouped. Click Group button. Select Ratio as Member/Reference. Check that Blank wells are solid color, or click Reference button to select reference well (*see* **Note 15**).

6. In Enter Sample Info window, enter description of each sample for appropriate sample number.

7. In Run Protocol window, select appropriate run conditions: Microsphere 50–100 per region, Sample timeout 120 s, run at High RP1 Target (*see* **Note 16**).

8. Click eject button to open tray. Place 96-well plate in tray and click start button to start analysis.

9. Bio-Plex/Luminex will display Median Fluorescent Intensity for each analyte.

10. In the Report table Window, display ratio to see signal to background ratios. Determine appropriate threshold signal to background ratio to define positive and negative samples (*see* Table 1).

3.5 MagPix

Perform adjust sample probe height, calibration, performance verification routines as described in operator's manual to ensure proper operation of instrument.

1. Open Protocols page. In the Protocols tab, click < create new protocol >.

2. Enter Assay Name, Version number, select microsphere number as 50, select qualitative for assay (*see* **Note 17**). Click < Next >.

Table 1
7-plex STEC serotyping immunoassay

Strain	O serogroup specific antibodies						
	O26	O45	O103	O111	O121	O145	O157
O26	**190.3**	1.4	1.4	1.6	1.2	1.3	1.4
O45	1.0	**53.3**	1.0	1.1	0.9	1.0	1.0
O103	1.0	1.0	**52.9**	1.0	0.8	1.0	1.0
O111	1.0	0.9	1.0	**60.6**	0.8	0.9	0.9
O121	1.2	1.0	1.1	1.0	**50.7**	1.1	1.0
O145	1.2	1.0	1.0	1.0	1.0	**78.9**	1.0
O157	1.2	1.1	1.2	1.1	1.2	1.2	**33.5**

STEC strains of the O serogroups indicated were grown overnight in Brain Heart Infusion Broth at 37 °C. Samples were diluted to an OD600 of 0.01 in Phosphate Buffered saline pH 7.4. Samples were then tested by Luminex immunoassay using O serogroups specific antibodies [3] conjugated to MagPlex microspheres and read on a Luminex 100 using Bio-Plex Manager 6.0 software. Results are presented as signal to background ratios for each analyte where background consisted of all immunoassay components except the analyte. Signal to background ratios > 3.0 are considered positive and are highlighted in *bold*

3. In the Analytes tab, click to highlight the appropriate microsphere region numbers. Enter analyte names for each microsphere region.

4. Open Batch page. Click on Create < New Batch from existing protocol > and select appropriate protocol.

5. Enter Batch name. In the Plate Layout tab, assign wells to be analyzed.

6. Insert 96-well plate in MagPix and click < Run Batch > when ready.

7. Median Fluorescent intensities will be displayed for each analyte.

4   Notes

1. Luminex microspheres have proven to be an extremely versatile tool. Here we discuss Luminex immunoassays where antibodies are coupled to Luminex microspheres, but assays can also be designed to investigate receptor ligand interactions or enzymatic assays by using proteins of interest [4]. Furthermore, analogous to immunoassay, multiplexing of nucleic acid hybridization assays may be accomplished by coding microspheres with oligonucleotides that bind to biotinylated complimentary sequences [5]. While such molecular assays are

often faster to develop, because they do not require generation of antibodies, immunoassays report on the presence of actual protein products. In bacteria the correlation between possessing a gene and expressing the respective protein is often good, if imperfect. But in eukaryotic systems gene regulation makes protein expression phenotype vary wildly in response to environmental variables.

2. MagPix uses fewer microspheres per analysis than the flow cytometry instruments, and analyses may be negatively affected by excess microspheres. This can make optimization of MagPix assays somewhat more difficult. However, because MagPix does not rely on lasers, which must be maintained in perfect alignment, the MagPix is a more rugged instrument, less sensitive to movement or vibration. MagPix also requires use of superparamagnetic microspheres (MagPlex) whereas the flow cytometry instruments can use either paramagnetic (MagPlex) or polystyrene (MicroPlex).

3. Calculating a median fluorescent intensity of the 50–100 microspheres per region minimizes the effects of carryover of microspheres from well to well. It also smoothes out variations between microspheres, essentially combining the data from 50 to 100 separate measurements. Although the method specifies using 2,500 or 5,000 beads for the assay, only 50–100 are actually counted. This allows for substantial losses during sample handling, including possible aggregation of beads.

4. Users have various options of Luminex microspheres to choose from. Here we describe the superparamagnetic Magplex microspheres that can be easily separated out of solution by applying a magnetic field. This facilitates coupling antibodies to microspheres and improves recovery during wash steps. MicroPlex microspheres are carboxylated polystyrene beads that can be conjugated with the same chemistries. For polystyrene MicroPlex microspheres, separate microspheres by centrifuging at $\geq 8{,}000 \times g$ for 1–2 min instead of applying magnetic field.

5. CAUTION! NaOH is corrosive! Refer to MSDS and use proper safety precautions when handling.

6. An alternative coupling buffer is 0.05 M MES pH 5.0, (2[N-morpholino]ethanesulfonic acid). Weigh 2.44 g of MES. Bring up to 200 mL with dI water. Adjust pH to 5.0 with 5 N NaOH. Bring up to 250 mL with dI water.

7. Detector antibodies can be biotinylated using EZ-Link Sulfo-NHS-LC-Biotin (Thermo Scientific Pierce Protein Biology Products) or equivalent biotinylation kit.

8. Alternatively, one can use the Bio-Plex Amine Coupling Kit (Bio-Rad Laboratories) and follow the kit instructions.

9. Prolonged exposure of microspheres to ambient light may result in photobleaching of the internal dyes and misclassification of microspheres by Luminex instruments during analyses. In Bio-Plex Manager software, photobleaching can be detected by examining the bead classification histogram. Photobleached microspheres will appear below and to the right of proper bead gate. Prolonged exposure of SAPE to light may result in photobleaching of reporter molecule which may result in low signal or poor sensitivity.

10. For MagPix assays use 25 µL working microsphere mixture and 25 µL PBS–1 % BSA per well (a total of 2,500 microspheres per bead region per test)

11. Alternatively one can use a Bio-Plex Pro Wash Station (Bio-Rad Laboratories) for automated washing of magnetic microspheres to reduce labor and variability between experiments.

12. The Luminex flow cytometry instruments are precision instruments that rely on precise laser alignment and sensitive optics. Follow manufacturer's instructions on instrument setup. Instrument should be in an environment of stable temperature 15–30 °C that does not vary more than 2 °C with a relative humidity <80 %. Ensure that instrument is installed on a secure bench with minimal vibrations from other instruments.

13. Here we describe Bio-Plex Manager software. Other instruments may use different software such as xPONENT. If using other software, follow the same run protocol as mentioned above.

14. Subsequent analyses using the same panel can select the saved panel name from the drop-down menu.

15. Here we describe a qualitative detection assay. For quantitative assays, a standard curve can be generated from the standards menu.

16. RP1 is an instrument setting to increase sensitivity, but with a lower dynamic range. Users can optimize low RP1 or high RP1 settings for each assay.

17. MagPix instruments can also perform quantitative assays. Enter information for multiple standards.

References

1. Hu H, Columbus J, Zhang Y et al (2004) A map of WW domain family interactions. Proteomics 4:643–655
2. Schröder C, Jacob A, Tonack S et al (2010) Dual-color proteomic profiling of complex samples with a microarray of 810 cancer-related antibodies. Mol Cell Proteomics 9:1271–1280
3. Clotilde LM, Bernard C IV, Hartman GH et al (2011) Microbead-based immunoassay for simultaneous detection of Shiga toxins and isolation of Escherichia coli O157 in foods. J Food Prot 74:373–379
4. de Jong LAA, Uges DRA, Franke JP et al (2005) Receptor-ligand binding assays: technologies and applications. J Chromatogr B 829:1–25
5. Lin A, Nguyen L, Lee T et al (2011) Rapid O serogroup identification of the ten most clinically relevant STECs by Luminex microbead-based suspension array. J Microbiol Methods 87:105–110

Chapter 12

Multiplex Immunoassay: A Planar Array on a Chip Using the MagArray™ Technology

Laurie M. Clotilde, Heng Yu, and M. Luis Carbonell

Abstract

Multiplexing is an important tool in assay development as it allows simultaneous detection of numerous analytes. Current platforms with the capability to multiplex are often complex and expensive. Here, we describe a low-cost planar array on a chip capable of simultaneously detecting up to 80 different analytes using the MagArray technology in as little as 10 min. This technology is easy to operate, has a small footprint, and is highly portable as it does not require any moving parts and/or microfluidics. This technology also allows the user to obtain a real-time read-out, which is very useful for analyzing complex sample matrices and for assessing cross-reactivity easily, or to monitor the dissociation of low affinity proteins during washes. The recommended sample volume for analysis is 100 μL after dilution, but as little as 20 μL can be measured if needed.

Key words Multiplex, Immunoassay, Proteins, Chip, Magnetic, MagArray

1 Introduction

Multiplex immunoassays allow simultaneous detection of various analytes within the same test sample. However, current platforms capable of multiplexing are often complex and expensive. Here, we describe a low-cost planar array on a chip capable of simultaneously detecting up to 80 different analytes using the MagArray MR-110 chip reader. Each chip is composed of 80 giant magnetoresistive sensors on which sandwich ELISA immunoassays are built with magnetic nanotags (MNT), an alternative to fluorescent or enzymatic labels [1]. This technology utilizes a magnetic nanoparticle technology derived from the computer disk drive industry for use in diagnostics and makes the MagArray platform an easy-to-operate (i.e., easy as plugging a USB drive into a computer), small (i.e., $22 \times 13.5 \times 11$ cm), portable system (i.e., less than 1 kg) with no moving parts and/or microfluidics. When compared to conventional ELISA [2], the MagArray system is capable of detecting analyte(s) (i.e., in this case carcinoembryonic antigen

Robert Hnasko (ed.), *ELISA: Methods and Protocols*, Methods in Molecular Biology, vol. 1318, DOI 10.1007/978-1-4939-2742-5_12, © Springer Science+Business Media New York 2015

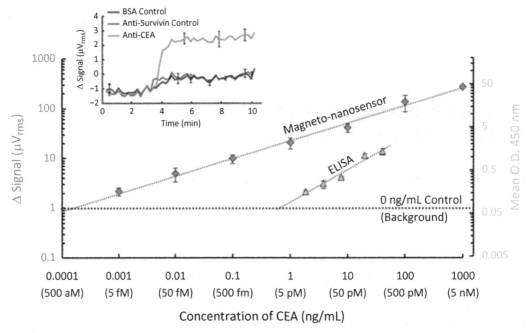

Fig. 1 Comparison of conventional ELISA to MagArray sensitivities for the biomarker CEA (figures taken from Gaster et al. [2])

[CEA]) at a much lower concentration and across a wider dynamic range (Fig. 1). In addition to superior performance in sensitivity, dynamic range, multiplexibility, and size, the MagArray system also possesses the following unique characteristics:

- Real-time read-out: All 80 sensors coated with the capture antibodies of interest are scanned every 4 s. The results are displayed as they are generated, thus allowing researchers to monitor binding with the MNT labels as it takes place. This special feature is extremely useful for "go/no go" decisions in a fast paced environment.

- Complex sample: Even optical interference caused by red blood cells is not a factor for the MagArray technology. While sensitivity is slightly less than serum, whole blood can be used as a suitable sample type as the chips are often insensitive to matrix effect [2]. This special feature should not be taken for granted and needs to be checked for every new analyte.

- Sequential addition of antibodies: It has long been recognized that cross-reactivity among the reagents in a multiplex assay is often a bottleneck in assay development. The open well system allows for detection antibodies to be sequentially added at any stage during the process [3]. Researchers can identify and isolate cross-reactivity issues in multiplex assays, as well as design assay procedures to circumvent certain cross-reactivity problems.

- No wash: The chip sensors only detect magnetic particles that have bound to the analytes of interest, but do not detect the bulk of unbound particles which float freely in the assay liquid. The net signal (i.e., bound particle fraction) is therefore accurately measured and equilibrates after several minutes. Thus, there is no need to wash before or after the addition of the MNT. This is of particular advantage when analyzing low affinity proteins that tend to get washed away during typical assay procedures.

- Small sample volume: Assays can be run using as little as a 20 μL sample after dilution, thus allowing researchers to run multiplex assays on minute samples from small animals such as mice or rats or on limited human samples that cannot be readily re-obtained.

Because of the advantages and characteristics listed above, the MagArray technology is an ideal platform of choice for detecting multiple analytes simultaneously.

2   Materials

2.1   Assay

1. Plastic chip cartridge (Fig. 2b) containing the coated chip (Fig. 2b) with antibodies of interest (*see* **Notes 1** and **2**), chip foam holder (Fig. 2c), and MNT can be purchased from MagArray (*see* **Note 3**).

2. Buffers:
   (a) Phosphate Buffered Saline (PBS).
   (b) Reaction Buffer (1 % Bovine Serum Albumin [BSA] in PBS) prepared by diluting BSA in PBS to 1 % (w/v) concentration and should be made fresh daily.
   (c) Rinsing Buffer (0.1 % BSA-PBS supplemented with 0.05 % Tween 20 [TPBS]) made by diluting BSA in TPBS (0.05 % Tween 20 in PBS) to 0.1 % (w/v) concentration and store at 2–4 °C.

3. Transfer pipette.

4. Scotch tape.

5. Sample of interest diluted to optimized concentrations using Reaction Buffer.

6. Detector antibodies of interest diluted to optimized concentrations using Reaction Buffer.

7. Rocking shaker.

8. Central vacuum system.

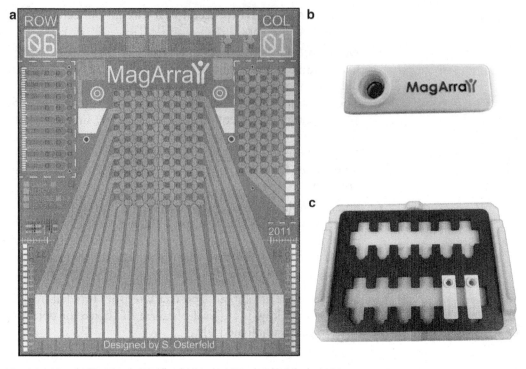

Fig. 2 (**a**) MagArray chip (10 × 12 mm), (**b**) cartridge, and (**c**) foam holder

2.2 Measurements

1. MagArray Chip Reader program (Fig. 3) and MagArray MR-110a reader (Fig. 4).

2.3 Disposal

1. Bleach.

3 Methods

3.1 Assay

Each chip has 8 built-in reference sensors (Fig. 2a), passivated and chemically isolated from the reaction well, that are used for establishing the level of electrical signal which is independent of assay chemistry during an assay (i.e., baseline or reference signal). The steps of the standard assay are described below, while the shortened steps for the express assay are described in the Notes (*see* **Note 4**). Also, a summary of the standard and express assay steps can be found in Figs. 5a, b.

1. Allow cartridges and samples to sit at room temperature for 30 min.
2. Dilute sample to desired concentrations in Reaction Buffer.
3. Add 100 μL of sample to the chip well (*see* **Note 5**).
4. Cover chip well with Scotch tape.

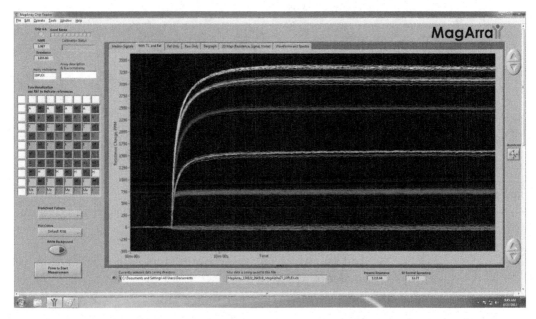

Fig. 3 MagArray Chip Reader program showing a 10-Plex immunoassay with five positives and five negatives

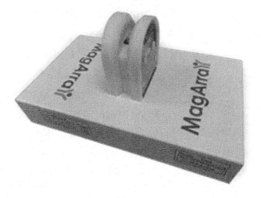

Fig. 4 MagArray MR-110a reader (22 × 13.5 × 11 cm; less than 1 kg)

5. Place chip cartridge into foam holder on Rocking Shaker and shake for 2 h at 350 +/− 20 rpm (*see* **Note 6**).

6. Prepare detection antibody to the desired concentrations in Reaction Buffer and allow it to warm to room temperature for 30 min.

7. Remove chip cartridge from Rocking Shaker and remove Scotch tape from chip well.

8. Wash the chips by aspirating out sample with central vacuum system by using a Transfer Pipette to fill the chip well with Rinsing Buffer and repeat washing **step 2** more times for a total of three washes.

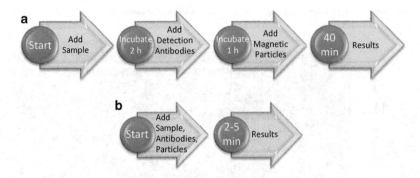

Fig. 5 Standard (**a**) and express (**b**) assay protocols

9. Add 100 µL of Detection Antibody Solution to the chip well (*see* **Note 5**).

10. Incubate for 1 h at room temperature (*see* **Note 6**).

3.2 Measurements

1. Open "MagArray Chip Reader" program on computer.

2. Enter assay run information: Operator Initials, Sample Number, and Run Number.

3. Input or load spotting pattern provided by MagArray.

4. Insert Plastic Chip Cartridge into the MagArray MR-110a reader.

5. Click on "Press to Start Measurement".

6. Wait until calibration is complete.

7. Wash the chip(s) by aspirating out detection antibody with central vacuum system by using a Transfer Pipette to fill the chip well with Rinsing Buffer and repeat washing **step 2** more times for a total of three washes.

8. Immediately add 100 µL of MNT solution (*see* **Note 5**).

9. Let measurement run for as short as 2 min from addition of MNT solution (*see* **Notes 6–9**).

10. Click on "STOP RECORDING" button in the MagArray Chip Reader program (*see* **Note 10**).

11. Data processing software is integrated in the data acquisition and the user can get a result sheet after stopping the assay.

3.3 Disposal

1. Remove chip cartridge from the MagArray MR-110a reader.

2. Fill chip well with bleach and allow to soak for at least 30 min.

3. Pour bleach into sink and allow chip to dry.

4. Put the chip cartridge into a designated container for disposal.

4   Notes

1. Make sure that the capture antibody solution does not have any surfactant. This will ruin your experiment. In addition, glycerol has also been known to decrease assay effectiveness.

2. Care should be taken not to scratch or let the face of chip come into contact with towels, pipette tips, or other materials. The sensor surfaces should never be touched.

3. MagArray's contact information can be found at www. MagArray.com and customized antibody-coated chips can be directly ordered.

4. For the express assay, all the reagents (i.e., sample, detector antibodies, and magnetic particles) are added at once, then the assay is measured right away and results obtained within 2–5 min. This was demonstrated to work with whole blood [2].

5. Make sure not to introduce any air bubbles when adding any reagents onto the chip as it might be detrimental to the quality of the results obtained.

6. The incubation times and temperatures can play a critical role in the assay optimization. The proposed incubation times and temperatures are the default commonly used, but once the assay is optimized for the reagents, consideration should be taken to shorten assay time by reducing incubation times and increasing or decreasing temperatures.

7. Problem: no signals from positive functional controls (Table 1).

8. Problem: low signals from positive functional controls (Table 2).

9. Problem: high signals from negative functional controls (Table 3).

10. The chip reader software automatically corrects for temperature variations during the assay and does not require the user

Table 1
Solutions when there are no signals from positive controls

Possible sources	Actions
Test station not working	Check connections
Chip not working	Check resistances
Bad positive probes	Check both positive probes and other sensors
Bad MNT solution	Check storage conditions/expiration date and/or order new particles

Table 2
Solutions for when there are low signals from positive controls

Possible sources	Actions
Bad probes	Replace with new antibody solution
Assay gone bad	Check other sensors

Table 3
Solutions for when there are high signals from negative controls

Possible sources	Actions
Insufficient washing	Rerun assay
Extremely high concentration of analyte	See the analyte concentration and titrate analyte even more
Detection antibody concentration too high	Optimize the concentration of detection antibodies
Probe denatured	Check other sensors

to activate it. Due to the complexity of this issue, the users are referred to Hall et al. [4].

If additional problems are encountered or any of the listed problems persist, please contact MagArray's technical support

Acknowledgement

MagArray team also includes Sebastian J. Osterfeld, R. Adam Seger, Alice Juang, and Shan X. Wang (Stanford University). The authors would like to acknowledge the support of the NCI SBIR Bridge Award to MagArray (R44CA165296) and the Center for Cancer Nanotechnology Excellence to Stanford University (U54CA151459).

References

1. Osterfeld SJ, Yu H, Gaster RS et al (2008) Multiplex protein assays based on real-time magnetic nanotag sensing. Proc Natl Acad Sci U S A 105:20637–20640

2. Gaster RS, Hall DA, Nielsen CH et al (2009) Matrix-insensitive protein assays push the limits of biosensors in medicine. Nat Med 15:1327–1332

3. Gaster RS, Hall DA, Wang SX (2010) Autoassembly protein arrays for analyzing antibody cross-reactivity. Nano Lett 11: 2579–2583

4. Hall DA, Gaster RS, Osterfeld SJ et al (2010) GMR biosensor arrays: correction techniques for reproducibility and enhanced sensitivity. Biosens Bioelectron 25:2177–2181

Chapter 13

Lateral Flow Immunoassay

Kathryn H. Ching

Abstract

Lateral flow immunoassays (LFIAs) are a staple in the field of rapid diagnostics. These small handheld devices require no specialized training or equipment to operate, and generate a result within minutes of sample application. They are an ideal format for many types of home test kits, for emergency responders and for food manufacturers and producers looking for a quick evaluation of a given sample. LFIAs rely on high quality monoclonal antibodies that recognize the analyte of interest. As monoclonal antibody technology becomes more accessible to smaller laboratories, there has been increased interest in developing LFIA prototypes for potential commercial manufacture. In this chapter, the basics of designing and building an LFIA prototype are described.

Key words Lateral flow, Immunochromatographic test strip, Rapid diagnostics, Antibodies, Gold nanoparticles

1 Introduction

Lateral flow immunoassays (LFIAs), also known as immunochromatographic strip tests, first emerged in the commercial market in the 1970s with the development of home pregnancy test kits [1]. These user friendly devices required no specialized training or invasive sampling, and gave users a qualitative answer within minutes of assay initiation. In vitro diagnostic device makers have since applied this technology to a wide array of analytical targets including for the identification of markers of infectious disease and toxic compounds, and for monitoring of metabolites indicative of drug use or the presence of disease [2, 3].

While LFIAs are simple and straightforward to operate for the user, their construction is complex, requiring a number of different solid materials and sophisticated biochemical reagents, the details of which are discussed here. At its core every LFIA depends on a labeled, mobile reagent and an antibody or analyte immobilized on the analytical membrane. LFIAs can be designed in two different formats, the direct format, which is essentially a sandwich ELISA (Fig. 1a),

Robert Hnasko (ed.), *ELISA: Methods and Protocols*, Methods in Molecular Biology, vol. 1318,
DOI 10.1007/978-1-4939-2742-5_13, © Springer Science+Business Media New York 2015

a Direct LFIA (sandwich ELISA)   **b** Competitive LFIA

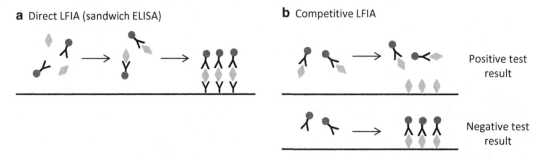

Positive test
result

Negative test
result

Fig. 1 (**a**) In the direct LFIA format, a labeled detector antibody moves through the analytical membrane with the analyte of interest. The antigen–antibody complex is captured by an immobilized, analyte-specific antibody, resulting in a *colored line*. (**b**) In the indirect format, the analyte of interest is immobilized on the analytical membrane. If analyte is present in the sample, it will bind the detector antibody, and the complex will flow past the immobilized analyte (*upper panel*). If there is no analyte in the sample, the detector antibody will bind the immobilized analyte, resulting in a *colored line* (*lower panel*)

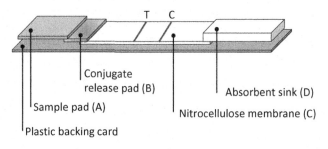

Conjugate
release pad (B)

Sample pad (A)   Absorbent sink (D)

Plastic backing card   Nitrocellulose membrane (C)

Fig. 2 Schematic of a lateral flow device

and the competitive format, which is an inhibition assay (Fig. 1b). The competitive format is generally developed for the detection of small molecules and will not be discussed here, but it should be noted that many of the same materials discussed below can also be employed in the competitive LFIA format. In the sandwich format, the focus of this chapter, a detector antibody, specific for the analyte of interest, is labeled with a visually detectable marker, such as gold nanoparticles or dyed polystyrene microspheres (these are sometimes erroneously called "latex beads") and dried onto a conjugate release pad (Fig. 2). The conjugate release pad overlays the analytical membrane, usually composed of nitrocellulose cast onto a plastic backing. A second analyte-specific antibody is immobilized on the analytical membrane. An antibody that recognizes the F_c region of the detector antibody is also separately immobilized on the analytical membrane, and serves as a control to indicate that the test components are working. At the distal end of the membrane, a thick pad, referred to as the "absorbent sink" soaks up sample fluid, allowing continued capillary flow through the membrane.

To initiate the assay, the sample is applied to the sample pad and flows into the conjugate release pad, rehydrating the detector antibody. The sample and detector antibody interact as they flow into the analytical membrane. If the analyte of interest is present, it binds the labeled detector antibody. As the complex moves up the membrane, it passes the immobilized analyte-specific antibody, which recognizes and binds it, resulting in a colored line. The control antibody recognizes and captures the F_c portion of the detector antibody, also resulting in a colored line which serves as a control. Here we describe the basics of developing a lateral flow assay first by briefly discussing some of the important considerations in material selection, followed by a step-by-step protocol we developed in our laboratory and have used successfully to build a highly sensitive and selective LFIA that could detect and distinguish between two serotypes of *Clostridia botulinum* that cause human illness [4].

2   Materials

Although all LFIAs are made up of the same basic test components, materials must be selected based on the individual requirements of the assay. The flow properties of the analytical membrane and the absorptive capacity of the distal sink, for example, can vary widely depending on the material chosen. As an example, GE Whatman's Immunopore membranes have relatively slow capillary rise times, which increases the interaction time between test components and analyte as the test runs. In contrast, while also highly sensitive, their AE line of nitrocellulose membranes have much faster rise times, and are more appropriate for viscous samples or samples with a high particle load. Deciding the particular requirements of the LFIA to be built and gaining a working knowledge of the materials available from different manufacturers is critical to designing a test with high sensitivity and specificity.

1. *Backing card:* The backing card serves as a platform for assembly of the different components of the test and is coated with a diagnostic grade pressure sensitive adhesive (PSA), which bonds materials quickly at room temperature with light pressure. PSAs manufactured for in vitro diagnostics (IVDs) are specially formulated so they will not interfere with test components (*see* **Note 1**). Protective release liners covering the card are typically manufactured with backsplits so the user can uncover certain portions of the adhesive as the test is assembled (*see* **Note 2**).

2. *Analytical membrane:* The analytical membrane will contain immobilized capture antibodies and serve as the test platform (*see* **Note 3**). Nitrocellulose membranes are the most widely

used in LFIA for a number of reasons. They have high protein binding capacity, true capillary flow characteristics and are relatively low cost. The production process for nitrocellulose membranes varies greatly between manufacturers. Choosing a supplier with experience in the manufacture of diagnostic grade membranes is critical to achieving reproducible results for an LFIA (*see* **Note 4**). As the market for LFIAs has increased, manufacturers have developed membranes with varying flow characteristics and sensitivities, and made considerable strides in improving CVs for capillary rise time, giving users more consistent results. In general, the capillary rise time of a membrane is inversely related to the sensitivity of the assay. In an ideal situation, the detector antibody has a fast on rate for its analyte, and binds immediately upon sample addition and rehydration. In reality, the time that the sample spends within the conjugate release pad before making contact with the analytical membrane is critical to assay sensitivity. An analytical membrane with a fast capillary rise time may not allow adequate time for detector antibody–analyte interaction, thereby decreasing the sensitivity of the assay. Application of capture antibodies to the analytical membrane should be performed using a quantitative dispensing system, such as the BioDot Quanti BioJet (Fig. 3). This non-contact liquid dispensing system allows the user to control the amount of capture antibody applied to the membrane, which can greatly influence assay sensitivity (*see* **Note 5**).

3. *Sample pad*: The sample pad receives the sample to be tested, but can also play an active role in preparing the sample for analysis. For example, a glass fiber sample pad can remove particulate

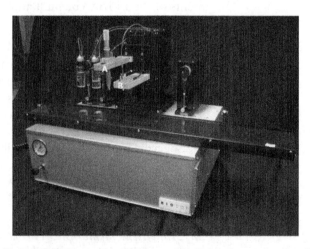

Fig. 3 BioDot XYZ Dispensing Platform. (**a**) AirJet for conjugate dispense. (**b**) BioJet for immobilization of capture antibodies

matter from a sample, thereby improving flow and assay performance. If the pH of a sample needs to be adjusted prior to analysis, the sample pad can be pretreated with assay buffer prior to its assembly in the device. Sample pad pretreatment can also include the addition of blocking materials (e.g., synthetic polymers such as PVP or PVA), detergents and surfactants, all of which can improve assay sensitivity and sample flow.

4. *Conjugate release pad*: The conjugate release pad contains dried, labeled detector antibody. Ideal materials for this component will hold the conjugate stably over the storage life of the test, and allow even rehydration and even release into the analytical membrane. Before the conjugate is applied, pads must be pretreated, either by the manufacturer or the developer prior to use. Pretreatment with blocking reagents and surfactants is typically done by immersion of the material in the pretreatment solution, followed by drying. Application of the conjugate itself can also be achieved by immersion, but this is not recommended. Ideally, conjugate is dispensed using a quantitative method, such as the BioDot AirJet Quanti dispensing system (Fig. 3). The system is similar to an artist's airbrush, aerosolizing the conjugate. This system allows the user to control the amount of conjugate applied to the pad, and more importantly, dispenses the conjugate in an even layer on the surface of the pad. Release of the conjugate from pads prepared with such a dispenser is typically more efficient and higher than pads treated by immersion.

5. *Absorbent Sink:* As the assay runs, the absorbent sink soaks up the sample fluid as it reaches the distal end of the strip. The sink is typically made from material with high absorptive capacity and is critical to preventing backflow of the sample which can result in high background signal and even false positives. GE Life Sciences manufactures a number of different sinks made of mixtures of glass fiber and cotton. The sink greatly affects the flow rate of the assay, as different materials have different wicking rates and absorptive capacities. When selecting a sink, one should consider the volume of sample to be applied.

6. *Antibody Pair:* A lateral flow device functions much like a sandwich ELISA, using an antibody pair to detect the target antigen. High-quality antibodies are the key to assay sensitivity, and choosing between monoclonal, polyclonal, or recombinant antibody will depend on the specific needs of your assay. Capture and detector antibody pairs should be identified by screening in an ELISA format (*see* **Note 6**). The chosen detector antibody is labeled with gold nanoparticles (see below), dyed polystyrene microspheres or a fluorescent marker and is dried down in the conjugate release pad. The capture antibody is immobilized on the nitrocellulose (see below).

7. *The antibody label:* Gold nanoparticles or dyed polystyrene spheres are typical labels for detector antibodies in LFIAs. Antibody labeling with 40 nm gold nanoparticles is probably the most well-known strategy and can be accomplished by two methods: passive adsorption onto the particles or direct conjugation (*see* **Note 7**). Gold particles can be produced in any lab by citrate reduction [5]. Producing a batch of particles with uniform size is more difficult, but is essential to the successful development of an LFIA. Many manufacturers of LFIA test components, such as Diagnostic Consulting Network, now offer small batches of gold sol at relatively low cost with particles of uniform size and at a specific optical density. This large volume of gold sol gives the user a significant amount of material with which to evaluate different test components, but does require a blocking step to prevent the gold surface from binding nonspecifically to other test components. Alternatively, covalent labeling kits are now available. Innova Biosciences InnovaCoat® GOLD, for example, works to directly conjugate antibodies via lysine residues to 40 nm gold particles. This process requires less antibody than passive adsorption and also does not require an extra blocking step because the gold surface is protected from nonspecific protein binding by a proprietary coat. More recently, Innova introduced a directed labeling kit which orientates Fab' fragments on the surface of the nanoparticles and an Fc specific conjugation kit for orientated labeling of IgGs, effectively increasing the sensitivity of the assay.

8. *Sample Buffer:* While not a structural component of an LFIA, the composition of the sample buffer must be considered. The pH of the buffer affects the performance of the antibody. Consider buffers with a neutral pH and low ionic strength, such as PBS or borate. Buffers. Surfactants such as Tween or Triton X-100 can be added to the running buffer, and can improve the flow rate. These reagents may also affect the affinity of the analyte for the antibody, so their use must be carefully considered. Blocking reagents can be added to the sample buffer as well. In general, it is best to use low concentrations of several different blocking reagents rather than one reagent at a high concentration.

3   Methods

3.1   Detector Antibody Labeling with Colloidal Gold

The structure of colloidal gold is a core of elemental gold surrounded by a shell of negative charge. The surface of gold nanoparticles has both hydrophobic and electrostatic characteristics. In its native state, the negative charges on the surface of the gold nanoparticles repel one another, and a colloidal suspension is maintained.

Proteins are adsorbed onto the surface through hydrophobic forces. Labeling proteins with gold nanoparticles requires two determinations: (1) the optimal pH for adsorption to occur and (2) the optimal protein concentration to completely coat the surface of the gold. If the optimal pH is not determined, electrostatic interactions between the protein and sol will result in precipitation of the reagents. If the surface is not sufficiently coated, the gold will precipitate out in the presence of any salts that are part of the assay's buffer system.

3.2 Determination of Optimal pH for Adsorption

All pH determinations of gold sol should be performed using litmus paper as the gold will damage electrodes. The optimal pH at which adsorption occurs for a particular protein will be the pH at which electrostatic interactions are minimized and hydrophobic interactions prevail (*see* **Note 8**).

1. Prepare 0.5 mL aliquots of gold sol with increasing pH values (increments of pH 0.5 using 0.2 M K_2CO_3 should suffice). The range should be around the isoelectric point of the ligand of interest. Mouse IgGs typically have a pI of 8.5.

2. Add these suspensions to 50 μL of a 1 mg/mL aqueous solution of the IgG of interest.

3. The smallest pH value at which flocculation, as described above, *does not occur* is the optimal pH for conjugation (*see* **Note 9**).

3.3 Determination of the Minimal Amount of Ligand Required for Conjugate Stability

The addition of salt to a suspension of colloidal gold will interfere with the repulsive charges between the gold particles, resulting in flocculation of the gold as described above. If the surface of the colloidal gold is sufficiently "protected" by adsorbed molecules, the addition of high concentrations of salts will have no effect on the colloid. This property can be exploited to determine the minimal amount of ligand required to stabilize the colloid.

1. Adjust the pH of colloidal gold and the antibody to be conjugated to the pH as determined above with 0.2 M K_2CO_3.

2. Prepare a range of antibody dilutions (1–50 μg/mL) in aqueous solution.

3. Pipette 100 μL of diluted antibody into a tube. Add 0.5 mL gold to each tube. Incubate 10 min at room temperature (The mixture should remain pinkish).

4. Add 0.5 mL 10 % NaCl to each tube. If the gold has been sufficiently coated with antibody, the addition of salt should not affect the suspension. If an inadequate amount of antibody has been added, the gold will precipitate out, turning the solution a purplish color. The tube with the lowest antibody concentration that remains pink after the addition of salt represents the minimal amount of antibody required to stabilize the gold in suspension (*see* **Note 10**).

3.4 Conjugation of ms IgG to 40 nm Colloidal Gold

1. Pipette 1 mL of colloidal gold into a small beaker.

2. Adjust the pH as determined above using 0.2 M K_2CO_3.

3. Add 10 % more antibody than the calculated amount to the gold.

4. Incubate the mixture for 10 min at room temperature.

5. Add BSA to a concentration of 1 %.

6. Swirl gently.

7. Transfer the mixture to a microfuge tube and spin at $15,000 \times g$ for 30 min in a fixed-angle rotor centrifuge.

8. Carefully aspirate the clear supernatant. Non aggregated gold-conjugated IgG will pool at the bottom of the microfuge tube. The dark pellet on the side of the tube is aggregated gold that has not been coated with antibody.

9. Slowly pipette off the pooled conjugated gold-IgG and transfer to a clean microfuge tube.

10. Mix the conjugate with 0.5 mL 20 mM Tris, pH 8.2 with 1 % BSA. Centrifuge as before.

11. Aspirate the supernatant and repeat **step 10**.

12. Aspirate the supernatant.

13. Suspend the conjugate in storage buffer (20 mM Tris, pH 8.2; 40 % glycerol; 1 % BSA; 0.01 % TX-100).

14. Store at 4 °C.

3.5 Immobilization of Capture Antibodies Using a BioJet Quanti Liquid Dispensing Non-contact System

1. Capture antibodies should be affinity purified and dialyzed in PBS at neutral pH.

2. Cut a 300 mm strip of Immunopore FP membrane (25 mm width).

3. Lay the strip down on the BioDot platform, aligning the edge of the membrane with the lip of the platform. Turn on vacuum to hold strip in place.

4. Prepare test capture antibody dilutions ranging from 0.5 to 2.5 mg/mL in PBS containing 3 % methanol (*see* **Note 11**).

5. Dispense test antibody 12 cm distal from the edge of the membrane at varying concentrations at a rate of 1 μL/cm in 40 nL drops (*see* **Note 12**). Mark the right edge of the strip where the capture antibody was laid down for future reference with a ball point pen.

6. Dispense control capture antibody 4 cm distal from the test antibody at 1 mg/mL at a rate of 1 μL/cm in 40 nL drops. Again, mark the right edge at the end of the dispensed line.

7. Use a test tube rack to hold the membrane (like a file in a file holder) and dry the membrane in a forced air drying oven for 20 min.

8. Block the membrane by immersion in blocking buffer. You will need to determine the optimal blocking buffer for your system. Again, the best way to determine this is to test a number of different reagents. Most blocking reagents used in LFIA are applied at very low concentrations. For example, PVA and PVP are typically used at a concentration between 0.1 and 5 %. Fish gelatin, casein, and Tween are also other commonly used reagents. Block for 20–30 min at room temperature (*see* **Note 13**).

9. Dry in a forced air drying oven for 20 min.

3.6 Preparation of the Conjugate Release Pad

Pretreatment of the conjugate release pad is necessary to ensure its stability during storage and for optimal release upon assay initiation. Hydrophilic polymers in low concentrations (i.e., <1 %) are effective reagents to achieve good release.

1. Cut a 6 mm × 300 mm length of Fusion5 (GE Healthcare). Pretreat the conjugate release pad by immersion in pretreatment solution. Again, you will need to determine what is best for your system.

2. Dry the pad in a forced air drying oven for 20 min.

3. Place the dried conjugation pad on the BioDot platform, aligning the bottom edge with the lip of the platform.

4. Dispense conjugate at a rate of 1 μL/cm in 40 nL drops with the Y-axis set at 3 mm. The dispensed conjugate will have uneven edges.

5. Dry the pad for 20 min in a forced air drying oven for 20 min, again using the test tube rack. Note that the side that was sprayed does not look the same as the side facing the platform.

3.7 Assembly of the Lateral Flow Device

1. Remove the center backsplit from the plastic backing card.

2. Wearing gloves carefully align the prepared analytical membrane (i.e., containing immobilized antibodies and completely blocked and dried) along the bottom edge of the exposed adhesive. Replace the backsplit over the nitrocellulose and apply gentle, even pressure to the membrane. Allow the membrane to rest for 20 min.

3. Remove the remaining backsplits.

4. Affix the absorbent sink with an approximately 2 mm overlap with the nitrocellulose.

5. Affix the conjugate release pad with an approximately 2 mm overlap with the nitrocellulose. Be sure that the side that was sprayed is the side that is facing up.

6. Affix the sample pad (Standard 14, GE Healthcare) over the conjugate release pad with an approximately 2 mm overlap.

7. Allow the assembled device to rest for 20 min.

8. Cut strips in 5 mm width using a guillotine cutter (*see* **Note 14**).

9. Place strips in cassettes (Diagnostic Consulting Network).

10. Store at room temperature with desiccant.

4 Notes

1. Other types of adhesives will contain solvents that can leach out into test components and interfere with assay stability and performance. Do not attempt to substitute other types of commercial adhesives.

2. Lohmann Corporation provides a range of choices for precut adhesive backing cards and can also custom manufacture cards for customers.

3. Nitrocellulose membranes for lateral flow can be purchased with and without a plastic backing. Although they may be more expensive, membranes cast onto a plastic backing are sturdier and easier to handle.

4. Whatman (GE Healthcare) and EMD Millipore both manufacture a wide array of nitrocellulose membranes for LFIA with varying flow characteristics and surface properties. Whatman and Pall Corporation are good sources for other LFIA components, including conjugate release pads and absorbent sinks.

5. The volume of antibody dispensed per drop directly correlates with the width of the capture antibody line. Empirical testing of this variable can demonstrate its effect on assay sensitivity.

6. It is recommended that as many capture-detector antibody pair combinations as possible are screened in the ELISA format, and then rank ordered by performance. You may find that the pair that performs best in ELISA is not the best pair for LFIA, or you may observe that an antibody that is a weak capture by ELISA may perform better as a capture in the LFIA format. Collect as much information as possible about your antibodies in the ELISA format; this systematic approach will save time in the end.

7. Both methods have their merits in development of LFIAs. Gold sol can be purchased in relatively large quantities at low cost. Having such a large stock of label available is helpful when identifying optimal antibody pairs or testing other test components such as blocking reagents and surfactants. Antibodies labeled using a kit designed to optimize coating will most likely not suffer from as many background or nonspecific binding issues.

8. This value has been determined for many commonly labeled proteins, and has typically been observed to be approximately

0.5 pH units higher than the adsorbed protein's isoelectric point (pI). At this point, the net charge on the protein of interest is around zero, and electrostatic interaction is minimized.

9. Naked gold sol less than 100 nm in diameter appears reddish in color. When precipitation of the gold occurs, the solution will appear purplish-gray. You may see smaller black precipitate in solution.

10. Spectroscopy can also be used to assess the change in color. Measure absorbance between 510 and 550 nm.

11. The addition of methanol to the capture antibody at a concentration from 1 to 3 % v/v has been shown to improve the resolution of the test and capture lines. Capture antibodies can be stored at 4 °C for several weeks. You will most likely begin to see a gradual decline in capture ability, however, as time passes.

12. Always wear gloves when handling nitrocellulose.

13. A good strategy to test different blocking buffers is to lay down a long strip with control and test capture antibodies (e.g., 300 mm), then cut the strip into smaller sections and immerse in different buffers. Be sure to notch one edge of each smaller strip so you know the orientation (a small notch in the upper right hand corner will suffice).

14. If such a cutter is not available, a paper cutter with a rotary blade can suffice for making LFIA prototypes. The edges of the nitrocellulose, however, will be damaged slightly and effect the flow of sample through the test strip. To minimize this effect, use a sharp blade and cut with a swift, even stroke. You may have to run the blade more than once over the strip; try to minimize the number of times you do this.

References

1. Leavitt SA (2003) A timeline of pregnancy testing. The Office of NIH History http://history.nih.gov/exhibits/thinblueline/timeline.html

2. O'Farrell B (2009) Evolution in lateral flow-base immunoassay systems. In: Wong RT, Tse HY (eds) Lateral flow immunoassay. Springer, New York, pp 1–33

3. Posthuma-Trumpie GA, Korf J, van Amerongen A (2009) Lateral flow (immuno)assay: its strengths, weaknesses, opportunities and threats. A literature survey. Anal Bioanal Chem 393:569–582

4. Ching KH, Lin A, McGarvey JA et al (2012) Rapid and selective detection of botulinum neurotoxin serotype-A and -B with a single immunochromatographic test strip. J Immunol Methods 380:23–29

5. Yokota S (2010) Preparation of colloidal gold particles and conjugation to protein A, IgG, F(ab')(2), and streptavidin. Methods Mol Biol 657:109–119

Chapter 14

Immuno-PCR Assay for Sensitive Detection of Proteins in Real Time

Xiaohua He and Stephanie A. Patfield

Abstract

The immuno-PCR (IPCR) assay combines the versatility and robustness of immunoassays with the exponential signal amplification power of the polymerase chain reaction (PCR). Typically, IPCR allows a 10–1,000-fold increase in sensitivity over the analogous enzyme-linked immunosorbent assay (ELISA). This is achieved by replacing the signal-producing antibody–enzyme conjugate of an ELISA with an antibody–DNA conjugate that serves as a marker for PCR amplification. The amplification power of the PCR allows for the detection of even single molecules of nucleic acid templates, making it well suited for a broad range of applications. Here, we describe the application of an IPCR assay for detection of trace amount of antigens using ricin as an example.

Key words Enzyme-linked immunosorbent assay (ELISA), Immuno-PCR, Real-time PCR, Restriction enzyme digestion, Ricin, TaqMan master mix

1 Introduction

The IPCR technique was originally introduced in 1992 by Sano et al. [1]. The assay protocol has since been modified to improve the immobilization of the antigen and the assembly of the signal-generating immuno-complex, enabling quantitative readout and data analysis in real time [2–6].

The basic protocol of an IPCR assay includes four parts: immobilization of the antigen; assembly of the immuno-complex; signal amplification by real-time PCR; and data analysis. Immobilization of antigens can be achieved in two ways: (a) attachment of the antigen to the surface of a microplate by passive adsorption; (b) oriented immobilization of the antigen using a specific capture antibody [7]. The immuno-complex has been assembled in four ways: (a) the biotinylated detection antibody is bridged by streptavidin to a biotinylated DNA marker; (b) the biotinylated detection antibody is tagged by an anti-biotin–DNA conjugate; (c) the detection antibody is directly conjugated with the DNA marker;

Robert Hnasko (ed.), *ELISA: Methods and Protocols*, Methods in Molecular Biology, vol. 1318, DOI 10.1007/978-1-4939-2742-5_14, © Springer Science+Business Media New York 2015

(d) the detection antibody is conjugated with streptavidin, and then reacted with the biotinylated DNA marker [4, 7]. PCR amplification of signal has been approached in two ways: (a) the whole IPCR process is completed in the same plate [8]. In this case, real-time PCR is carried out directly in the wells where the immuno-complex is assembled; (b) the whole IPCR is carried out in two different plates. The first plate is for assembly of the immuno-complex, and the second plate is for amplification of signal by PCR. For data analysis after the PCR, an automatic baseline correction is usually applied by the software of the instrument and the cycle thresholds (Ct) are calculated automatically. The amount of the target protein in each sample can be determined based on a standard curve plotted by the Ct values against the log concentrations of the target protein for linear correlation.

IPCR offers several advantages over conventional protein detection methods. First, the limit of detection is greatly improved compared to immunoassays [9–11]. Second, the sample volume required is very small. The high sensitivity of IPCR enables the analysis of sample sizes of less than 1 μL. This is of particular importance for studies where only limited volumes of samples are available [12]. Third, the assay is compatible with most complex biological matrices [8]. Owing to the high sensitivity of IPCR, the biological sample can usually be diluted, which significantly reduces the matrix effect. Fourth, the use of real-time PCR, rather than end point PCR, improves the quantitative accuracy of the assay.

Here, we introduce a sandwich IPCR assay. This assay uses a "sandwich" of antibodies to capture and detect a protein of interest as done in a sandwich ELISA, with an additional step using a DNA marker that binds to the detection antibody through an avidin–biotin interaction allowing for signal amplification by real-time PCR (Fig. 1).

The method takes advantage of the high affinity bond between biotin and streptavidin to form a streptavidinated antibody-biotinylated DNA complex. Because excess proteins and DNA can interfere with PCR, the DNA is made cleavable from the antibody complex by incorporating a BamHI restriction site at the 5′ end. After cleaving the DNA from the immuno-complex, an aliquot is transferred to real-time PCR tubes or 96-well plates containing a PCR master mix cocktail with primers and a probe with a fluorescent reporter. Throughout the PCR cycle, the real-time PCR cycler detects and records changes in the fluorescence signal during amplification. This amplification signal is used to calculate the cycle threshold (Ct) value. The Ct is defined as the number of cycles required for the fluorescent signal to cross the threshold (i.e., exceed background levels). Ct levels are inversely proportional to the amount of DNA in the sample such that the lower the Ct value, the greater the amount of DNA in the sample and, therefore, the greater the amount of target antigen. The DNA probe has a

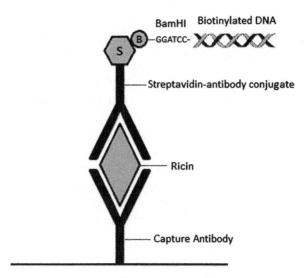

Fig. 1 Schematic representation of the Sandwich IPCR method, depicting the analytical complex on the surface of an assay well. The assay involves using a capture antibody, antigen (ricin), and streptavidin-conjugated detection antibody. The DNA marker is linked to the immuno-complex through a biotin–streptavidin interaction. *B* biotin, *S* streptavidin

fluorescent reporter at one end and a quencher of fluorescence at the opposite end of the probe. The close proximity of the reporter to the quencher prevents detection of its fluorescence until the 5′ to 3′ exonuclease activity of the Taq polymerase breaks the reporter–quencher proximity and thus allows emission of fluorescence, which can be detected upon excitation with a laser. An increase in the product targeted by the reporter probe at each PCR cycle therefore causes a proportional increase in fluorescence due to the breakdown of the probe and release of the reporter.

As with all immunoassays, the sensitivity of IPCR largely depends on the antibodies selected to bind and detect the target antigen. The sandwich IPCR requires two antibodies, each with a strong affinity to different epitopes of the antigen. A polyclonal antibody can be used as both the capture and detection antibody but the use of a monoclonal antibody for capture tends to provide more reproducible results due to the consistent and even coating across each well. It is recommended that sandwich ELISAs be carried out to determine the best antibody pair for each particular antigen before applying the antibodies to the IPCR method. The limit of detection (LOD) for IPCR is defined as the average Ct value of the negative controls (wells containing buffer or sample matrix only without any antigen) plus three times the calculated standard deviation. In order to calculate the standard deviation and, subsequently, the LOD, it is necessary to perform the assay with triplicates for each sample.

Using the procedures described here, we demonstrate that the sandwich IPCR can detect 10 pg/mL of ricin in chicken egg and bovine milk samples and 100 pg/mL in ground beef extracts. Comparable ELISA results were in the 1–10 ng/mL range [7]. Thus, IPCR affords sensitivity that is tenfold greater in the ground beef matrix, 100-fold greater in the milk matrix, and 1,000-fold greater in the egg matrix than the sensitivity obtained by ELISA (Table 1). This IPCR is also highly compatible with complex environmental matrices. When applied to 23 environmental samples including feces, feral swine colon, soil, and water from watersheds for detecting the presence of Shiga toxin 2 produced by Shiga toxin-producing *E. coli* (STEC), it demonstrated a 100 % sensitivity and specificity [13].

Table 1
Detection of ricin in liquid egg, milk, and ground beef extract

Method	Ricin Concn (pg/mL)	Avg C_T (SD) or A_{450} (SD)[a]		
		Liquid egg	Milk	Ground beef extract
Sandwich IPCR[b]	0	27.94 (0.01)	29.35 (0.02)	27.68 (0.11)
	10	26.78 (0.28)	28.21 (0.37)	27.94 (0.40)
	100	26.41 (0.24)	27.09 (0.43)	26.79 (0.03)
	1,000	25.11 (0.04)	24.03 (0.03)	25.97 (0.04)
	10,000	22.46 (0.30)	20.96 (0.01)	22.81 (0.19)
	100,000	19.63 (0.22)	18.23 (0.20)	20.00 (0.67)
	1,000,000	18.05 (0.12)	17.36 (0.09)	18.90 (0.22)
Sandwich ELISA[c]	0	0.39 (0.02)	0.40 (0.02)	0.38 (0.33)
	100	0.41 (0.01)	0.40 (0.01)	0.42 (0.01)
	1,000	0.44 (0.02)	0.67 (0.03)	0.73 (0.06)
	10,000	1.06 (0.00)	1.41 (0.04)	1.16 (0.03)
	100,000	2.13 (0.05)	2.24 (0.07)	2.16 (0.03)
	1,000,000	NA	NA	NA

[a]Values are C_T for sandwich IPCR and A_{450} for sandwich ELISA. *NA* not available
[b]LOD for sandwich IPCR: liquid egg and milk, 10 pg/mL; ground beef extract, 100 pg/mL
[c]LOD for sandwich ELISA: liquid egg, 10,000 pg/mL; milk and ground beef extract, 1,000 pg/mL

2   Materials

Prepare all solutions using ultrapure water (prepared by purifying deionized water to attain a sensitivity of 18 MΩ cm at 25 °C) and analytical grade reagents. Prepare and store all reagents at room temperature (unless otherwise indicated). Follow all waste disposal regulations when disposing of waste materials.

1. Reagent buffer: 50 mM boric acid, pH 9.5. Weigh out 0.309 g boric acid and add water and 1–5 M NaOH to 100 mL volume at pH 9.5. Sterilize by filtration and store in 5–10 mL aliquots at −20 °C.

2. Tris-buffered saline (TBS): 20 mM Tris-Cl, 150 mM NaCl, pH 7.5. Weigh out 8 g NaCl, 0.2 g KCl, and 3 g Tris Base and dissolve into 1 L water plus 1–5 M HCl to pH 7.5. Autoclave at 121 °C for at least 30 min to sterilize.

3. Bovine Serum Albumin–Tris-buffered saline (BSA–TBS): TBS containing 0.5 % (wt/vol) bovine serum albumin (BSA), 5 mM EDTA, and 0.2 % (wt/vol) NaN_3. Dissolve 1 g BSA, 0.4 g NaN_3, and 0.29 g EDTA into 200 mL TBS (*see* **Note 1**). Sterilize by filtration and store in 50 mL aliquots at −20 °C (*see* **Note 2**).

4. Tween/EDTA/Tris-buffered saline (TETBS): TBS containing 5 mM EDTA and 0.05 % (vol/vol) Tween 20. Weigh out 1.46 g EDTA and stir into 1 L TBS until dissolved completely. Stir in 0.5 mL Tween 20 until dissolved completely (*see* **Note 3**). Autoclave at 121 °C for at least 30 min to sterilize.

5. Reagent dilution buffer: Prepare from fresh BSA–TBS and TETBS in a 1:10 ratio. Mix 1 mL BSA–TBS with 9 mL TETBS (*see* **Note 4**).

6. Anti-ricin monoclonal antibody 1642 (USDA, Albany, CA).

7. Streptavidin-conjugated anti-ricin antibody: prepare using Lightning-Link Streptavidin Conjugation Kit (Innova Biosciences Ltd., Cambridge, UK) following the manufacturer's instructions: Mix 100 μL of 1 mg/mL anti-ricin polyclonal goat antibody (Vector Laboratories, Burlingame, CA) with 10 μL of LL-Modifier reagent and then add to vial containing 100 μg of lyophilized LL-streptavidin. Incubate the mixture for 3 h at room temperature (RT), and then add 10 μL of LL-quencher reagent. The conjugate can be used after 30 min or stored at 4 °C.

8. Biotinylated DNA marker: A mono-biotinylated DNA marker was prepared by PCR using the pUC19 plasmid as the template and the primer pair: pUC-bio (20) (5'-biotin-CCCG-GATCCCAGCAATAAACCAGCCAGCC-3') and F1 (5'-TAT GCAGTGCTGCCATAACCATGA-3'). Perform amplification

with Taqman Universal PCR Mastermix with an initial 95 °C denaturation for 10 min followed by 40 cycles of 95 °C for 15 s and 60 °C for 1 min (*see* **Note 5**).

9. BamHI restriction endonuclease and buffer 3.1 (New England BioLabs).

10. 96-well V-bottom microtiter plate (USA Scientific, Orlando, FL) (*see* **Note 6**).

11. Adjustable speed orbital plate shaker such as the Barnstead/ Lab-Line Titer Plate Shaker, or similar.

12. Incubator set to 37 °C.

13. Multichannel pipette and filter tips (*see* **Note 7**).

14. 1.5 mL low-adhesion microfuge tubes (USA Scientific) (*see* **Note 8**).

15. 0.2 mL Temp Assure PCR 8-tube flex-free strips with individually attached, optically clear flat caps (USA Scientific) or similar Real-time PCR tubes or plates (*see* **Note 9**).

16. TaqMan Universal PCR 2× Mastermix (Applied Biosystems)

17. Primers:

F (5′-CCATAACCATGAGTGATAACACTGCT-3′)

R (5′-CGATCAAGGCGAGTTACATGATC-3′)

18. Probe (5′-Fam-ACCGAAGGAGCTAACCGCTTTTTTGC AC-Tam-3′)

19. Real-Time PCR cycler (e.g., Mastercycler Eppendorf Realplex) (*see* **Note 10**).

3 Methods

Carry out all procedures at room temperature unless otherwise specified. Plate washes are carried out on an oscillating plate shaker, set to a low shaking speed (*see* **Note 11**). Wear gloves for all steps and change them frequently to avoid contamination. Keep workspace clean and free of DNA, antigens, and other sources of contamination by wiping down regularly.

3.1 Immunoassay

1. Dilute anti-ricin monoclonal antibody 1642 to 4 μg/mL in reagent buffer and coat a 96-well microtiter plate with 30 μL of antibody dilution per well (*see* **Note 12**).

2. Incubate covered plate overnight at 4 °C (*see* **Note 13**).

3. Wash the wells three times for 1 min with 150 μL of TBS (*see* **Note 14**).

4. Block non-adsorbed sites with 150 μL of BSA–TBS per well and incubate for 1 h (*see* **Note 15**).

5. Wash wells twice for 30 s and twice for 4 min with 150 µL of TETBS.

6. Prepare tenfold serial dilutions of ricin in TBS and add 30 µL per well of each dilution and incubate for 1 h (*see* **Note 16**).

7. Wash wells as in **step 5**.

8. Add 30 µL per well of streptavidin-conjugated anti-ricin polyclonal antibody at a final concentration of 80 ng/mL in reagent dilution buffer and incubate at 37 °C for 30 min.

9. Wash wells as in **step 5**.

10. Add 30 µL per well of biotinylated DNA marker at 0.5 ng/µL in TETBS and incubate for 30 min. Keep any remaining dilution on ice for the positive PCR control.

11. To remove unbound DNA, wash wells four times for 30 s and three times for 4 min with TETBS, followed by five times for 1 min with TBS.

12. Detach bound DNA from the immuno-complex by incubating the wells with 30 µL of restriction buffer containing 1 unit per well of BamHI for 2 h at 37 °C (*see* **Note 17**).

13. Use 6 µL of digested DNA as a template in real-time PCR (20 µL reaction volume) (*see* **Note 18**).

3.2 Real-Time PCR

1. Prepare 1× PCR mastermix as follows, multiplying the volume by the number of samples to be analyzed (*see* **Note 19**):

TaqMan Master Mix (2×)	10 µL
10 µM primer F	0.6 µL
10 µM primer R	0.6 µL
10 µM Probe	0.5 µL
Water	2.3 µL
	14 µL

2. Aliquot 14 µL PCR mastermix to real-time PCR tubes with caps, one per sample, plus one each for positive and negative PCR controls.

3. Add 6 µL of digested DNA as a template. For the positive control sample, add 1 µL of the DNA marker dilution at 0.5 ng/µL and 5 µL of water. For the negative control, add 6 µL of water to the master mix. Close all caps. Wipe caps with precision wipes to remove dust before placing in PCR cycler (*see* **Note 20**).

4. Run PCR program: 95 °C 10 min (95 °C 15 s, 62 °C 1 min), ×40 cycles, 4 °C, hold. Use a heated lid. Set the volume to 20 µL and background calibration to IPCR tubes (*see* **Note 21**). Set FAM as the fluorophore and tetramethylrhodamine as the quencher.

5. Use Realplex software to calculate baseline and cycle threshold (Ct) values (*see* **Note 22**).

4   Notes

1. BSA–TBS includes the preservative NaN_3 which can cause harm via contact with skin, eyes or upon ingestion. Use proper PPE when preparing and handling this solution.

2. BSA–TBS can be frozen and thawed repeatedly but should remain on ice throughout the assay procedure.

3. Tween is very viscous and sticky and therefore needs to be measured precisely and dissolved completely into solution to get an accurate final concentration.

4. Reagent dilution buffer should be made fresh and kept on ice during the assay and any excess discarded after use.

5. A BamHI restriction site was included in the pUC-bio primer to allow removal of the DNA marker from the immuno-complex. The resulting PCR product should be about 340 bp when run on an agarose gel for analysis. Purify the PCR product using a QIAquick PCR Purification Kit (Qiagen, Valencia, CA) and determine the concentration by Nanodrop or using a UV–visible spectrophotometer.

6. You may substitute TopYield strips or other thermally stable, small-welled plate with a high-binding capacity. If using Top Yield strips, increase the wash and block buffer volumes to 200 μL per well.

7. Filter tips should be used to prevent cross-contamination. Be careful not to touch the tips to the wells of the plate while pipetting and change them between each washing and between pipetting different reagents or antigens into the wells.

8. For preparation of antigen dilutions, low adhesion tubes are used to minimize nonspecific binding of protein, allowing greater accuracy and sensitivity when performing IPCR.

9. If using a PCR plate, it must be sealed with optically clear tape and covered with a compression pad (rubber mat with holes, aligned properly for measurement of fluorescence) when placed in the PCR cycler.

10. PCR can also be done using a conventional PCR cycler followed by analysis of DNA concentrations by gel electrophoresis. However, quantitative real-time PCR has the advantages of shorter handling time and greater reproducibility.

11. The shaker should be set to a speed of two or three, such that the plate is oscillating swiftly but the wash solution is not splashing from the wells. Alternatively, an automatic plate washer may be used with the following protocol: aspirate, wash 6×150 μL, with aspiration following each wash.

12. The concentration of capture antibody for coating plates can vary but should be in the range of 0.5–5 μg/mL for best results.

13. Cover with plastic wrap or plate-sealing tape to prevent evaporation from wells. Plates can be left at 4 °C for up to 3 days with little or no effect on assay outcome.

14. For each wash step, use a multichannel pipette to add wash buffer to wells, then place on the orbital shaker for the time specified. Repeat as specified.

15. Alternate blocking buffers/concentrations can be substituted if high background is observed in a particular application of IPCR that may not be compatible with BSA or requires a higher concentration of blocking agent.

16. The dilutions should be in the range of 0.01 pg/mL to 100 ng/mL. The optimal range will vary based on the strength of antibodies used. When analyzing samples with unknown antigen concentration, be sure to include a full set of standards for comparison and quantification.

17. Use a buffer suitable for BamHI, such as buffer 3.1 or 2.1 from New England BioLabs, and dilute it to 1× with sterile nuclease-free water prior to adding the restriction endonuclease. The endonuclease typically is supplied at a concentration of 20 units/μL and should be diluted to yield 1 unit per 30 μL. Cover plate with a tight-sealing tape or film to prevent evaporation.

18. Remaining digested DNA can be kept at 4 °C overnight if the experiment needs to be repeated the next day.

19. For short-term storage (less than 30 min), keep mastermix on ice in the dark to protect the probe against degradation.

20. Any dust particles or other contamination on the PCR tubes will block the measurement of fluorescence and skew the results.

21. Follow instructions in the real time PCR cycler manual for calibrating the tubes or plates that will be used for the PCR step.

22. If random signals and high error are observed, check PCR wells for background fluorescence and contamination. Also check PCR tubes for evaporation and ensure heated lid is working. If positive signals are observed in the negative controls, check all PCR reagents for contamination.

References

1. Sano T, Smith CL, Cantor CR (1992) Immuno-PCR: very sensitive antigen detection by means of specific antibody-DNA conjugates. Science 258:120–122

2. Lind K, Kubista M (2005) Development and evaluation of three real-time immuno-PCR assemblages for quantification of PSA. J Immunol Methods 304:107–116

3. Niemeyer CM, Adler M, Pignataro B et al (1999) Self-assembly of DNA-streptavidin nanostructures and their use as reagents in immuno-PCR. Nucleic Acids Res 27:4553–4561

4. Niemeyer CM, Adler M, Wacker R (2007) Detecting antigens by quantitative immuno-PCR. Nat Protoc 2:1918–1930

5. Shan J, Toye P (2009) A novel immuno-polymerase chain reaction protocol incorporating a highly purified streptavidin-DNA conjugate. J Immunoassay Immunochem 30: 322–337

6. Zhou H, Fisher RJ, Papas TS (1993) Universal immuno-PCR for ultra-sensitive target protein detection. Nucleic Acids Res 21: 6038–6039

7. He X, McMahon S, McKeon TA et al (2010) Development of a novel immuno-PCR assay for detection of ricin in ground beef, liquid chicken egg, and milk. J Food Prot 73: 695–700

8. Spengler M, Adler M, Jonas A et al (2009) Immuno-PCR assays for immunogenicity testing. Biochem Biophys Res Commun 387: 278–282

9. Adler M, Wacker R, Niemeyer CM (2008) Sensitivity by combination: immuno-PCR and related technologies. Analyst 133:702–718

10. Barletta JM, Edelman DC, Constantine NT (2004) Lowering the detection limits of HIV-1 viral load using real-time immuno-PCR for HIV-1 p24 antigen. Am J Clin Pathol 122: 20–27

11. Fischer A, von Eiff C, Kuczius T et al (2007) A quantitative real-time immuno-PCR approach for detection of staphylococcal enterotoxins. J Mol Med (Berl) 85:461–469

12. Barletta J, Bartolome A, Constantine NT (2009) Immunomagnetic quantitative immuno-PCR for detection of less than one HIV-1 virion. J Virol Methods 157:122–132

13. He X, Qi W, Quinones B et al (2011) Sensitive detection of Shiga Toxin 2 and some of its variants in environmental samples by a novel immuno-PCR assay. Appl Environ Microbiol 77:3558–3564

Chapter 15

In Situ Proximity Ligation Assay (PLA)

Sonchita Bagchi, Robert Fredriksson, and Åsa Wallén-Mackenzie

Abstract

In situ proximity ligation assay (PLA) is a method to identify physical closeness of proteins, where a signal will only be produced if the two proteins are closer than 40 nm, in tissue section or cell cultures. Modifications of the PLA method can also be used to increase specificity or sensitivity of standard immunohistochemistry protocols.

Key words Proximity ligation assay (PLA), Immunohistochemistry, In situ, Oligonucleotides, Rolling circle replication, Fluorescence

1 Introduction

The Proximity ligation assay (PLA) is an antibody-based method to detect biomolecules and their physical proximity, which can in principle be any molecules that can be recognized by antibodies. The technique was first introduced in 2002 with an assay that was able to detect zeptomoles (10^{-21} mol) of platelet derived growth factor (PDGF) in solution phase [1]. Subsequently the assay was modified to detect also cytokines [2] and then the assay was adapted to detect and visualize proteins, protein complexes, and protein modification in situ via the in situ PLA [3]. Currently, reagents for this assay are available as a commercial kit (http://www.olink.com/) primarily intended for detecting proximity between two proteins, although the method can be extended to many other applications.

The principle for detection of proximity between two targets requires two antibodies, one directed against each of the targets under investigation. An outline of the method is presented in Fig. 1a, b (left panel). The two antibodies are conjugated either directly to special PLA probes (Fig. 1b), which are target-specific antibodies modified by attaching short DNA oligonucleotides, or they are unlabeled but then must be produced in different species (Fig. 1a). In the case where the primary antibodies are produced in different

Robert Hnasko (ed.), *ELISA: Methods and Protocols*, Methods in Molecular Biology, vol. 1318,
DOI 10.1007/978-1-4939-2742-5_15, © Springer Science+Business Media New York 2015

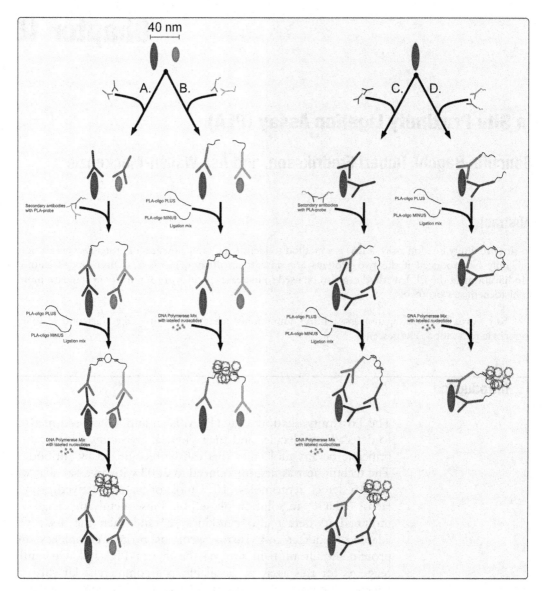

Fig. 1 Schematic diagram illustrating the principle of the PLA. The *left panel* illustrates measurement of protein proximity or interaction while the *right hand panel* illustrates detection of a single protein with two antibodies

species, two general secondary antibodies with oligonucleotides pre-attached can be used. The two PLA probes, called PLA oligo PLUS and PLA oligo MINUS, have stretches of nucleotides which are complementary to two standard oligonucleotides that are included in the ligation step. These two oligonucleotides will hybridize to the PLA oligo PLUS and MINUS if they are close, and allow for ligation to occur, inducing the two oligonucleotides to form a circle. The last step is the amplification, which will produce many copies of the complements of this circle using the DNA polymerase Phi29 pol in a process called Rolling Circle Replication (RCR).

These copies are detected by hybridizing fluorescence-labeled nucleotides, to produce signals that can be detected using standard fluorescent microscopy.

The PLA technology can also be used to increase specificity and/or sensitivity in standard immunohistochemical analyses, *see* Fig. 1c, d (Right panel). In the case of increased specificity, the two antibodies are directed against different epitopes of the same protein. This requires both antibodies to bind specifically to the correct target protein to produce a signal; while false binding, where only one of the antibodies binds the correct target will not be detected. This setup increases specificity significantly because the specificity of two independent antibodies is used. This can be performed using either PLA-probes linked directly to the primary antibodies (Fig. 1d) or by utilizing general secondary PLA antibodies as secondary markers (Fig. 1c). Again, the approach in Fig. 1c requires the two primary antibodies to be raised in different species.

If only one primary antibody is available for a given target, PLA can still be of value to increase sensitivity, but not specificity. This procedure is also based on two secondary antibodies, with PLA oligonucleotides PLUS and MINUS attached, although both are directed against different epitopes within the same target protein antibody. This will allow for the amplification step to produce many fluorescent signals in the RCR process to increase sensitivity, but the specificity will be solely dependent on the single primary antibody. In fact, any false signals will be strongly amplified, and therefore, this approach relies on having a very specific primary antibody to provide meaningful results.

The ability to detect and visualize small quantities of proteins, as well as various interactions between proteins and different post-translational modifications, is crucial for early diagnosis and subsequent early intervention of different diseases. With the increased knowledge of the molecular basis of many conditions, the vision of an increasingly personalized medicine is becoming a reality [4]. Several studies have employed PLA for screening various kinds of human tumors and carcinomas and here we present a few examples. One recent study describes how PLA has been implemented for the screening of serum/plasma material for identification of potential biomarkers, in order to determine treatment and treatment outcome [5]. In another study, this technique was used to identify receptor tyrosine kinase activation, demonstrated by phosphorylation status, in sample preparations derived from people suffering from choroid plexus tumors [6]. A third study showed in situ interaction in human glioblastoma samples between specific proteins of a known signaling pathway previously shown to interact in vitro [7]. Neuroscience is an additional field where the colocalization and interaction of proteins is of high interest, both from a more clinical point of view as well as preclinical.

In a recent study, the subcellular colocalization of a newly identified transporter protein of the SLC superfamily with presynaptic marker proteins such as synaptophysin was validated in cell-line-based material by PLA following an immunohistochemical approach [8]. Finally, with a direct aim at improving clinical diagnosis, neuroscientists evaluated PLA for detection of Aβ-aggregates, and by comparing this technique with the sandwich ELISA found a 25-fold increase in sensitivity [9], while in another study, scientists used the PLA for in situ detection of interaction between the major component of Lewy bodies, α-synuclein, a hallmark protein complex found in patients with Parkinson's disease, with the dopamine transporter protein [10]. In summary, although the PLA was invented no more than some 10 years ago, its applications have been seen in many different areas and including both preclinical and clinical research. Our own experience of the technique is positive and we recommend new users to follow the protocol carefully and to include all necessary controls (*see* Subheading 3.1) to enable proper analysis of the end result.

2   Materials

1. The Duolink II fluorescence kit (orange detection reagents, Olink Biosciences, Sweden) can be used to run in situ proximity ligation assay technology (PLA) on fixed cells or paraffin-embedded tissue sections (*see* **Note 1**).

2. IgG class primary antibodies (not included in the kit) specific to each proteins whose interactions are to be detected, are crucial for the success of each PLA. The antibodies could be either monoclonal or polyclonal. The primary antibodies are required to be optimized beforehand with immunohistochemical (IHC) and/or immunofluorescence (IF). Same concentrations and conditions are recommended to be used for PLA.

PLA probe PLUS reagents in this kit are stored at 4 °C and the components are as follows

3. Blocking solution (1×) for blocking of the sample.

4. Antibody diluent (1×) to be used to dilute both primary antibodies and the PLA probes.

5. PLA probe anti-Rabbit/Mouse/Goat PLUS (5×) is secondary antibody conjugated to oligonucleotide PLUS. Depending on the species used to raise the primary antibody, the probe is designed to bind to it in a specific manner.

6. The Blocking solution and the Antibody diluent are to be used without further dilution. The PLA probes must be diluted 1:5 in 1× Antibody diluent before use.

PLA probe MINUS reagents in this kit are stored at 4 °C and the components are as follows

7. Blocking solution (1×) for blocking of the sample.

8. Antibody diluent (1×) to be used to dilute both primary antibodies and the PLA probes.

9. PLA probe anti-Rabbit/Mouse/Goat MINUS (5×) is secondary antibody conjugated to oligonucleotide MINUS. Depending on the species used to raise the primary antibody, the probe is designed to bind to it in a specific manner.

10. The Blocking solution and the Antibody diluent are to be used without further dilution. The PLA probes must be diluted 1:5 in 1× Antibody diluent before use.

Detection Reagents must be stored at –20 °C and include the following

11. Ligation (5×) contains oligonucleotides that bind to the PLA probes and other components for ligation (except the enzyme 'ligase').

12. Ligase (1 U/μl) is the enzyme for ligation.

13. Amplification Orange (5×) contains all components needed for Rolling Circle Amplification (except the enzyme 'Polymerase') and oligonucleotide probes labeled with fluorophore that hybridize to the Rolling Circle Amplification product.

14. Polymerase (10 U/μl) is the enzyme for amplification.

15. Duolink In situ Wash Buffers A and B. These specific buffers are used during all washing steps as indicated in the protocol. They are bought in powder form in a pouch. The entire content of the pouch has to be dissolved in 1,000 ml of high purity water. The stocks can be stored at 4 °C for long-term storage. Buffers A and B can be kept at room temperature for maximum of 1 week.

16. Duolink In Situ Mounting Medium with DAPI. This medium is used to prepare the glass slides prior to microscopic imaging to preserve PLA signals without immediate fading or diffusion and can be stored at 4 °C.

17. Slides and coverslips.

18. Pipettes (ranging from 1 to 1,000 μl).

19. Grease pen.

20. Humidity chamber.

21. 37 °C incubator.

22. Freeze-block for enzymes.

23. Staining jars.

24. Shakers.

25. Fluorescence microscope with proper filter (Cy3 for detection with Orange detection kit).

26. Camera and software for image acquisition.

27. Duolink ImageTool for analysis and quantification of PLA signals.

3 Methods

3.1 Primary Antibodies

For each PLA between two proteins, primary antibodies must be obtained against each of them, and they must be produced in different species. Otherwise, they cannot be distinguished by the PLA probes. PLA probe PLUS and PLA probe MINUS recognize two individual antibodies depending on their host species. *It is possible, however, to run PLA between antibodies raised in the same species using Duolink* In Situ *Probemaker kit. This product enables conjugation of PLA oligonucleotide arms directly to primary antibodies. Duolink* In Situ *Probemaker PLUS and Duolink* In Situ *Probemaker MINUS should be used (instead of PLA probe PLUS and PLA probe MINUS, respectively) to differentiate between two primary antibodies attached to two proteins of interest.*

3.2 Controls

For proper evaluation of results, it is important to include controls for each sets of assay. As a positive control, two proteins known to be in close proximity or interacting should be chosen. This will verify success of the PLA procedure. Negative controls can be biological or technical. For biological negative control, a cell or tissue can be chosen where one or both of the target proteins are not expressed. This will account for the specificity of the antibodies used as well as the accuracy of execution of the procedure. For a technical negative control PLA may be run while omitting one or both of the primary antibodies. This will show the background signals. Too many signals in this control might indicate insufficient washing steps and failure to perform the procedure correctly.

3.3 Proximity Ligation Assay

All reagents except the enzymes should be thawed at the room temperature and vortexed before use. *The enzymes should be kept cold (–20 °C) at all times* and to be added to the reaction mixes immediately before use. The 5× stocks should be diluted with high purity water prior to each use. All incubations must be performed without coverslips in a preheated humidity chamber. 40 μl of reaction volume will cover 1 cm² area of sample, delimited with grease pen. Open droplet reactions are to be used. The entire reaction area must be covered with reagents/solutions at all times.

Day 1

1. Deposit samples on glass slides and pretreat with fixatives, antibody retrieval and permeabilization.

2. Add one drop of blocking solution per 1 cm^2 area of sample (*see* **Note 2**).

3. Incubate the slides in a preheated humidity chamber for 30 min at 37 °C (*see* **Note 3**).

4. Dilute primary antibodies to suitable concentrations in the Antibody Diluent (*see* **Note 4**).

5. Tap off the blocking solution (*see* **Note 5**).

6. Add primary antibody solutions to each sample.

7. Incubate the slides in a humidity chamber overnight at 4 °C (*see* **Note 6**).

Day 2

8. Dilute two PLA probes 1:5 in Antibody Diluent. For 40 μl reaction, add 8 μl of PLA probe PLUS stock and 8 μl of PLA probe MINUS stock to 24 μl of Antibody Diluent (*see* **Note 7**).

9. Tap off the primary antibody solutions (*see* **Note 5**).

10. Wash the slides 2×5 min with 1× Wash Buffer A in a staining jar with minimum volume of 70 ml on a shaker with gentle orbital shaking (*see* **Notes 8, 9** and **12**).

11. Add PLA probe solutions.

12. Incubate the slides in a preheated humidity chamber for 60 min at 37 °C (*see* **Note 3**).

13. Dilute the Ligation stock 1:5 in high purity water. For 40 μl reaction, add 8 μl of 5× Ligation stock into 31 μl of high purity water (*see* **Note 7**).

14. Tap off the PLA probe solution from the slides (*see* **Note 5**).

15. Wash the slides 2×5 min with 1× Wash Buffer A under gentle agitation (*see* **Notes 8, 9** and **12**).

16. Remove the Ligase from the freezer using a −20 °C freezing block. Then add Ligase to the Ligation solution from **step 13** at 1:40 dilution (for 40 μl reaction, add 1 μl of Ligase to 39 μl of Ligation solution) and vortex (*see* **Notes 10** and **11**).

17. Add the Ligation–Ligase solution to each sample.

18. Incubate the slides in a preheated humidity chamber for 30 min at 37 °C (*see* **Note 3**).

Light-Sensitive Reagents: Work in Reduced Light from Now on

19. Dilute the Amplification stock 1:5 in high purity water. For 40 μl reaction, add 8 μl of 5× Amplification stock into 31.5 μl of high purity water (*see* **Note 7**).

20. Tap off the Ligation–Ligase solution from the slides (*see* **Note 5**).

21. Wash the slides 2×2 min with 1× Wash Buffer A under gentle agitation (*see* **Notes 8, 9** and **12**).

22. Remove the Polymerase from the freezer using a –20 °C freezing block. Then add Polymerase to the Amplification solution from **step 19** at 1:80 dilution (for 40 μl reaction, add 0.5 μl of Polymerase to 39.5 μl of Amplification solution) and vortex (*see* **Notes 10** and **11**).

23. Add the Amplification–Polymerase solution to each sample.

24. Incubate the slides in a preheated humidity chamber for 100 min at 37 °C (*see* **Note 3**).

25. Tap off the Amplification–Polymerase solution from the slides (*see* **Note 5**).

26. Wash the slides 2×10 min in 1× Wash Buffer B (*see* **Notes 8, 9** and **12**).

27. Wash the slides in 0.01× Wash Buffer B for 1 min (*see* **Note 13**).

28. Dry the slides at room temperature in the dark (*see* **Note 14**).

29. Mount the slides with coverslips using minimal volume of Duolink In Situ Mounting Medium with DAPI. Avoid trapping air bubbles between the slide and the coverslip.

30. Seal the edges with nail polish.

31. Leave the slides in dark for 15 min (*see* **Note 15**).

3.4 Imaging and Analysis of PLA Signals

1. Image using a fluorescence or confocal microscope with Cy3 filter (when Duolink Orange detection kit is used) for detection of PLA signals and DAPI filter for the nuclear staining. Z-stacked images must be acquired in order to capture all the signals as well as to be able to count them using Duolink ImageTool software (*see* **Note 16**). An example of a PLA image of a mouse brain section can be seen in Fig. 2a, with the corresponding negative (no probe) control in Fig. 2b.

2. Duolink ImageTool can be used for objective quantification of PLA signals. Raw imaging data can be imported directly from the four major microscope vendors (Olympus, Leica, Nikon, and Zeiss) as well as tiff and jpg files.

3. After the images are imported, the nuclei are automatically detected. It is possible to adjust their size manually. The average cytoplasm size is estimated and threshold for identification of signals is assigned. By using this software, it is possible to record either the number of signals and cells per image using average measurements, or to designate each individual signal to a specific cell using single cell analysis. The results can then be exported to Microsoft Excel and further used for analysis and evaluation.

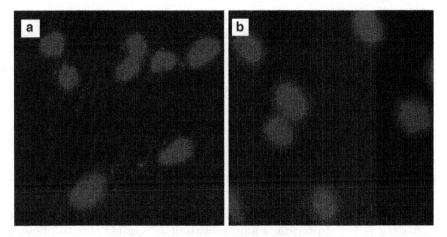

Fig. 2 Example of a PLA image showing a mouse brain section hybridized with antibodies against two synaptic proteins (**a**) and the corresponding negative (no probe) control (**b**)

4. Evaluation and representation of the data can be executed in any graph making program. One can use histograms or Pie diagrams to exhibit how interaction between two proteins might vary depending on sub-cellular localization, expression or functional modifications. The data set can be normalized using PLA signals acquired from two primary antibodies raised against the same protein but in different species. The following is an example. Protein X (detected using an antibody raised in rabbit) interacts with protein Y (detected using an antibody raised in mouse) as well as with protein Z (detected using an antibody raised in mouse). By counting the number of PLA signals, we can quantify and visualize the extent of the two interactions. However, the difference between these two interactions can depend on the level of expression of proteins Y and Z. Y may be more expressed than Z and hence more frequently interact with X and thus result in more PLA signals or vice versa. In order to control for this variation, two primary antibodies against Y (one raised in rabbit and one in mouse) can be used to produce PLA signals and then used to normalize the data set between X and Y by division X (rabbit) : Y (mouse)/Y (rabbit) : Y (mouse). Similarly, the ratio can be calculated for Z: X (rabbit) : Z (mouse)/Z (rabbit) : Z (mouse). This will produce the actual number of interactions between XY and XZ and hence can be fairly compared.

4 Notes

1. While using paraffin embedded sections, incomplete removal of paraffin can give high background. Ensure that all the solutions are fresh and the times are maintained during the deparaffinization steps.

2. Same blocking solution and wash buffer (e.g., PBS or TBS) as used previously in immunohistochemistry or immunofluorescence during optimization, can be used during Day 1 of PLA procedure in order to maximize binding of primary antibodies.

3. Preheat the humidity chamber at 37 °C each time prior to any incubation.

4. If any antibody diluent other than the one included in Duolink In situ kit is used, the PLA probes must also be diluted in the same diluent. In that case, the PLA probe mixture must be incubated at room temperature for 20 min before adding to the samples.

5. Always keep the reaction area moisten, but try to tap off the previous solutions as well as possible. Try to obtain the same residual volume on each slide as this can affect reproducibility.

6. The incubation time with primary antibodies can be adjusted depending upon individual antibodies.

7. Do not store diluted PLA probes or diluted reagents.

8. Always bring Wash Buffers A and B to room temperature before use.

9. Ensure sufficient washing with gentle agitations, but never exceed the time recommended for washing.

10. The concentrations of Ligation mix and Amplification mix must be accurate.

11. Keep the enzymes on a –20 °C freezing block at all times. Add the enzymes immediately before adding the mix to the samples. Vortex and mix after addition of enzyme each time.

12. Use only Duolink In situ Wash Buffers A and B for washing during the detection steps.

13. The 1 min washing step with 0.01× Wash Buffer B is crucial. Do not wash for more than 1 min.

14. Let the slides dry well before mounting. Keep them in dark.

15. Wait minimum 15 min before analyzing the slides under microscope.

16. After imaging, the slides can be stored at –20 °C for future analysis.

Acknowledgements

The authors thank Prof. Ulf Landegren at Uppsala University for constructive feedback during the preparation of this manuscript. Work by Bagchi and Fredriksson is supported by Swedish Research Council, The Swedish Brain Foundation, The Swedish Society for Medical Research, The Novo Nordisk foundation, Åhléns foundation, Engkvist Foundation, Thurings Foundation for metabolic research, Gunvor and Josef Anérs foundation, and Tore Nilssons foundation, and work by Wallén-Mackenzie by The Swedish Research Council, The Swedish Brain Foundation, Parkinsonfonden, Åhléns Foundation and the Hållsten Research Foundation.

References

1. Fredriksson S, Gullberg M, Jarvius J, Olsson C, Pietras K, Gustafsdottir SM et al (2002) Protein detection using proximity-dependent DNA ligation assays. Nat Biotechnol 20:473–477

2. Gullberg M, Gustafsdottir SM, Schallmeiner E, Jarvius J, Bjarnegard M, Betsholtz C et al (2004) Cytokine detection by antibody-based proximity ligation. Proc Natl Acad Sci U S A 101:8420–8424

3. Soderberg O, Gullberg M, Jarvius M, Ridderstrale K, Leuchowius KJ, Jarvius J et al (2006) Direct observation of individual endogenous protein complexes in situ by proximity ligation. Nat Methods 3:995–1000

4. Blokzijl A, Friedman M, Ponten F, Landegren U (2010) Profiling protein expression and interactions: proximity ligation as a tool for personalized medicine. J Intern Med 268:232–245

5. Tsai CL, Koong AC, Hsu FM, Graber M, Chen IS, Cheng JC (2013) Biomarker studies on radiotherapy to hepatocellular carcinoma. Oncology 84(Suppl 1):64–68

6. Hofacre CL, Glisson JR, Kleven SH, Brown J, Rowland GN (1989) Evaluation of Pasteurella multocida mutants of low virulence. I. Development and pathogenicity. Avian Dis 33:270–274

7. Petri MK, Koch P, Stenzinger A, Kuchelmeister K, Nestler U, Paradowska A et al (2011) PTPIP51, a positive modulator of the MAPK/Erk pathway, is upregulated in glioblastoma and interacts with 14-3-3beta and PTP1B in situ. Histol Histopathol 26:1531–1543

8. Hagglund MG, Hellsten SV, Bagchi S, Ljungdahl A, Nilsson VC, Winnergren S et al (2013) Characterization of the transporter-B0AT3 (Slc6a17) in the rodent central nervous system. BMC Neurosci 14:54

9. Kamali-Moghaddam M, Pettersson FE, Wu D, Englund H, Darmanis S, Lord A et al (2010) Sensitive detection of Abeta protofibrils by proximity ligation–relevance for Alzheimer's disease. BMC Neurosci 11:124

10. Latge JP, Bouziane H, Diaquin M (1988) Ultrastructure and composition of the conidial wall of Cladosporium cladosporioides. Can J Microbiol 34:1325–1329

Chapter 16

Tyramide Signal Amplification for Immunofluorescent Enhancement

Lauren Faget and Thomas S. Hnasko

Abstract

Enzyme-linked signal amplification is a key technique used to enhance the immunohistochemical detection of protein, mRNA, and other molecular species. Tyramide signal amplification (TSA) is based on a catalytic reporter deposit in close vicinity to the epitope of interest. The advantages of this technique are its simplicity, enhanced sensitivity, high specificity, and compatibility with modern multi-label fluorescent microscopy. Here, we describe the use of a TSA kit to increase the signal of enhanced green fluorescent protein (eGFP) expressed under the control of *Slc17a6* regulatory elements in the brain of a transgenic mouse. The labeling procedure consists of 6 basic steps: (1) tissue preparation, (2) blocking of nonspecific epitopes, (3) binding with primary antibody, (4) binding with horseradish peroxidase-conjugated secondary antibody, (5) reacting with fluorescent tyramide substrate, and (6) imaging of the signal. The procedures described herein detail these steps and provide additional guidance and background to assist novice users.

Key words Enzyme-linked immunodetection, Tyramide signal amplification (TSA), Catalytic reporter deposit, Fluorometric, Oxidoreduction, Horseradish peroxidase (HRP), Immunohistochemistry (IHC), Fluorescence, Antibodies, Green fluorescent protein (GFP), Vesicular glutamate transporter (VGLUT2)

1 Introduction

Immuno-based enzyme-linked signal amplification methods have been used for decades to detect and localize low copy number protein, mRNA, and other small molecules or probes present in tissue by immunohistochemistry, in situ hybridization, western blot and ELISA. Earlier amplification methods, for example using biotinylated secondary antibodies and streptavidin-conjugated reporters, are based on the formation of layers or complexes of immunocytochemical reagents. Enzyme-base amplification methods instead rely on a catalytic reporter deposit (CARD) and can increase signal relative to conventional fluorescent probes by as much as 100-fold [1, 2]. Alkaline phosphatase (AP) and horseradish peroxidase (HRP) are the most commonly used enzymes

Robert Hnasko (ed.), *ELISA: Methods and Protocols*, Methods in Molecular Biology, vol. 1318,
DOI 10.1007/978-1-4939-2742-5_16, © Springer Science+Business Media New York 2015

conjugated to secondary antibodies for immunohistochemical detection [3–5]. Compared to AP, HRP is smaller, more stable, and less expensive than alkaline phosphatase and has a high turnover rate that allows for the rapid generation of strong signals [3, 6].

A primary consideration is to weigh the advantages of a fluorescent signal versus a chromogenic reaction product visible with simple bright-field optics. Indeed, HRP-mediated CARD can produce either a chromogenic or fluorometric reaction product depending of the substrate added; for example 3,3′-diaminobenzidine (DAB) or dye-coupled tyramide respectively. Although yielding a rapid dark brown chromogenic precipitate that is compatible with tissue dehydration, numerous counterstains, and is highly stable, DAB is a teratogenic compound that needs to be disposed as a biohazard. Fluorescent dye-coupled tyramide is safer and more amenable to multi-labeling procedures using fluorophores with distinct excitation/emission spectra.

TSA was developed in the early 1990s [4, 5] and uses HRP to catalyze the deposition of labeled tyramide molecules at the site of probe or epitope detection. Tyramide is converted by HRP into a highly reactive oxidized intermediate which binds rapidly and covalently to electron-rich tyrosine residues present in GFP or other proteins in close proximity to the epitope (Fig. 1).

TSA can therefore provide better spatial resolution compared to other HRP or AP-based methods where reaction products may diffuse from the sites of enzyme activity [7]. In addition to the direct TSA system where tyramide is conjugated directly to the fluorophore, modifications have been developed to further increase sensitivity by coupling tyramide to haptens, such as biotin or dinitrophenyl (DNP), which have multiple binding sites and can then be detected by reporter-bound streptavidin or antibodies [8]. For instance, biotinylated tyramide has proven useful to reveal various tissue antigens with high resolution by electron microscopy [9].

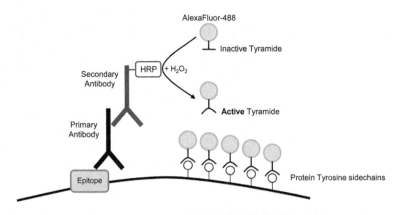

Fig. 1 Schematic illustrating Tyramide signal amplification strategy

The enhanced sensitivity provided by TSA allows one to decrease the concentration of primary antibody from 2 to 50-fold relative to classical approaches with reporter-conjugated secondary antibodies, generating a highly specific signal with low background signal [10]. Primarily used for detection of low copy number mRNA by fluorescent in situ hybridization (ISH) [11, 12], further uses of TSA include enhancement of low expression level protein signal by immunohistochemistry [13–16] and dual fluorescent labeling [7, 17]. In immunohistochemistry, TSA may also reveal otherwise undetectable proteins in subcellular compartments such as axons and dendrites [13, 14, 16].

We describe here the methods for the use of the TSA kit #12 from Invitrogen, though similar kits are available from other vendors (e.g., Perkin-Elmer). Though a variety of target species and fluorophores are available [18], this kit includes goat anti-rabbit secondary antibody coupled to HRP and Alexa Fluor-488-coupled tyramide—this green light emitting fluorophore is brighter and more photostable than earlier generation fluorophores such as fluorescein [1, 10]. As an example procedure we have stained coronal brain sections from a bacterial artificial chromosome transgenic (BAC-Tg) mouse line (GENSAT line FY115) expressing enhanced green fluorescent protein (GFP) under the control of *Slc17a6* regulatory elements to visualize neurons that express the vesicular glutamate transporter (VGLUT2) [19, 20]. Subsets of, presumably high expressing, VGLUT2+ neurons display sufficient intrinsic fluorescence for visualization in fresh tissue [21]. However, following aldehyde fixation, GFP fluorescence is significantly quenched and immunohistochemical procedures are required. Here we performed a side-by-side comparison of the signal obtained with a conventional method versus TSA-enhanced immunolabeling (Fig. 2). Using low concentrations of primary antibody, TSA generated less background signal, brighter cell bodies and revealed subcellular compartments that were otherwise subthreshold. TSA can therefore be an excellent strategy to conserve valuable primary antibodies and enhance signal-to-noise, particularly for high-background antibodies or low-copy number epitopes.

2   Materials

All solutions are prepared using double-distilled water (ddH$_2$O, 18 MΩ) and prepared and stored at room temperature unless indicated otherwise. Experiments were performed in compliance with the guidelines of the National Institutes of Health Guide for the Care and Use of Laboratory Animals and approved by the Institutional Animal Care and Use Committee at the University of California, San Diego.

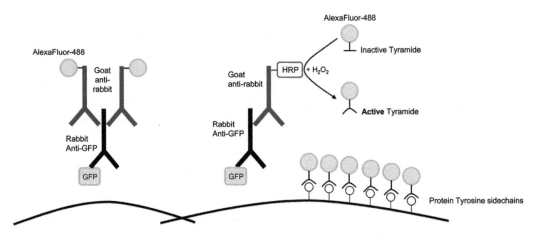

Fig. 2 Schematic comparing conventional immunofluorescence with tyramide signal amplification. Schematic comparing (**a**) conventional immunohistochemical labeling of a GFP epitope with a fluorophore-conjugated secondary antibody and (**b**) TSA. TSA uses the enzymatic activity associated with a HRP-conjugated secondary antibody to activate fluorophore-bound tyramide which accumulates near the epitope site. Activated fluorescent tyramide covalently binds to nearby tyrosine residues resulting in brighter signal while retaining subcellular specificity

Immunohistochemistry Materials

1. Sample preparation and fixation methods will vary by tissue type, species and epitope. For the example experiment described below we deeply anesthetized an 18-week-old BAC-Tg. VGLUT2-GFP mouse with ketamine (Ketaset, 100 mg/kg i.p.) and xylazine (AnaSed, 10 mg/kg i.p.), transcardially perfused with 10 mL of ice-cold phosphate-buffered saline (PBS) followed by 50 mL 4 % paraformaldehyde (PFA, Electron Microscopy Sciences, #19210) dissolved in PBS. The brain was harvested, post-fixed overnight at 4 °C in 4 % PFA, cryoprotected in 30 % sucrose (Fisher, # S2-212), frozen in superchilled (on dry ice) isopentane (Spectrum, # M1246) and stored at–80 °C. The brain was transferred to a cryostat chamber (Leica 3050) and allowed to equilibrate to–20 °C before cutting 30-µm sections, and sections were transferred to wells in a 48-well plate containing PBS plus 0.01 % sodium azide (*see* **Note 1**).

2. Small thin brushes: *Da Vinci* Ussuri red sable brushes no. 0, 1, and 2.

3. Pasteur glass pipettes melted and curved into a hook under a flame.

4. Non-coated 24-well culture plates, sterile, with lid, #662102, Cellstar.

5. Microscope slides, Superfrost Plus, pre-cleaned, $25 \times 75 \times 1.0$ mm, #22-034-979, Fisher.

6. Cover glass, thickness 1½, 22 × 50 mm, #2980-225, Corning.

7. Transfer pipets, #13-711-7 M, Fisher.

8. Petri dish, 5.5 in. diameter, #08-747 F, Pyrex 9. Polyethylene slide holder, #82024-526, VWR.

Immunohistochemistry Reagents

9. Polyclonal rabbit anti-green fluorescent protein, A11122, 2 mg/mL, Invitrogen. Upon receipt add equal volume 100 % glycerol (#AC158920025, Fisher) and store at–20 °C (stock concentration 1 mg/mL).

10. Donkey anti-rabbit conjugated to Alexa Fluor-488, #711-545-152, Jackson ImmunoResearch. Upon receipt reconstitute in lyophilized antibody in 0.5 mL of 50 % glycerol (1 mg/mL) and store at–20 °C. This antibody is used in the conventional immunostaining protocol.

11. Phosphate Buffered Saline, 10× solution, #BP399-1, Fisher. Prepare 1 L of PBS by diluting 10× PBS 1:10 in ddH$_2$O and store at 4 °C.

12. 0.2 % Triton X-100 in PBS. Prepare 1 L of PBS and add 2 mL of Triton X-100 (PBS-T); used for washes and incubation with antibodies in conventional immunohistochemistry method. Store at 4 °C.

13. Normal Donkey Serum (NDS), Jackson Immunoresearch, #017-000-121. NDS is used at a concentration of 4 % in PBS-T solution. PBS-T + 4 % NDS is used for blocking non-specific sites of labeling in the conventional immunostaining protocol. Prepare only the amount necessary for the experiment and use fresh.

14. Sodium azide, #BP922I-500, Fisher. To prepare preservation buffer for free-floating sections, add 100 mg of sodium azide to 1 L of PBS to obtain a final concentration of 0.01 % sodium azide. Store at 4 °C.

15. Mounting medium: Fluoromount-G, #0100-01, SouthernBiotech.

16. DAPI, 4′,6-diamidino-2-phenylindole, 20 mg/mL, #D1306, Invitrogen. DAPI binds strongly to A-T rich regions in DNA and is used as a nuclear counterstain. When bound to double-stranded DNA DAPI has a maximum emission wavelength at 461 nm (blue) [22]. DAPI is dissolved 1/2,000 (0.01 mg/mL) in Fluoromount-G mounting medium. Store at 4 °C, protected from light.

TSA Amplification Kit

17. In order to amplify the endogenous GFP signal we used the rabbit anti-GFP primary antibody, #A11122, from Invitrogen in association with the TSA Kit (Molecular Probes, #T-20922): Tyramide coupled to Alexa Fluor-488 (Component A).

Labeled tyramide is provided as a powder and dissolved in 150 μL of DMSO (Component B). Dissolve the powder in DMSO inverting the vial several times. To minimize freeze-thaw cycles, stock the solution in small aliquots of 5–10 μL, depending of the quantities required for individual experiments. Store aliquots at–20 °C, protected from light.

18. Dimethylsulfoxide, DMSO (Component B), 200 μL.

19. Horseradish peroxidase (HRP)-conjugated goat anti-rabbit (Component C), 100 μg. HRP-conjugated secondary antibody is reconstituted in 200 μL of PBS (0.5 mg/mL) (*see* **Note 2**). Filter PBS using a sterile 30 mm diameter and 0.22 μm PES membrane syringe filter (Bioexpress, #F-2690-9). Solution can be stored up to 3 months at 4 °C.

20. Blocking reagent (Component D), 3 g. Dissolve 10 mg of component D in 1 mL of PBS to prepare a 1 % blocking reagent solution (10 mg/mL). Blocking reagent solution should be prepared only when needed for immediate use. Store stock powder desiccated at–20 °C.

21. Amplification buffer (Component E), 25 mL (contains thimerosal at 0.02 %).

22. Hydrogen peroxide (30 %) stabilized solution in water (H_2O_2; Component F), 200 μL.

3   Methods

1. Immunostaining performed on 30 μm-thick fixed brain sections (*see* **Note 3**). Up to six sections are placed per well in a 24-well plate (*see* **Note 4**). It is important to not let brain sections dry during solution changes (*see* **Note 5**). Proceed with a thin brush or a smooth hooked glass Pasteur pipette to transfer sections from one well to another without damage. All incubation steps are performed in 1 mL/well with gentle agitation (35–50 rotations/min) and at room temperature unless otherwise specified (*see* **Note 6**).

2. Rinse to eliminate sodium azide residues: three 5–10 min rinses with PBS.

3. Permeabilize tissue with detergent to increase antibody penetration: one rinse with PBS-T for 5–10 min (*see* **Note 7**).

4. Peroxidase quenching to reduce background signal (*see* **Note 8**): stock solution is 30 % H_2O_2 in water (Component F). Dilute 100 μL of H_2O_2 stock solution in 2.9 mL of PBS to obtain 1 % H_2O_2 final solution. Incubate tissue in 1 % H_2O_2 for 20 min (*see* **Note 9**).

5. Remove residual H_2O_2: three 5–10 min rinses with PBS (*see* **Note 10**).

6. Block nonspecific binding sites: incubate with 1 % blocking reagent for 1 h (*see* **Note 11**). 1 % blocking reagent is prepared using 10 mg/mL Component D in PBS. Prepare the final volume necessary for blocking, primary antibody and secondary antibody incubations. If primary antibody incubation is planned overnight, prepare only the quantity necessary for blocking and the primary antibody incubation and prepare fresh blocking solution on day 2 for the secondary antibody incubation.

7. Primary antibody: dilute primary antibody in blocking solution and incubate 2 h at room temperature or over-night at 4 °C (*see* **Note 12**). We used a rabbit anti-GFP diluted in 1 % blocking reagent solution (*see* **Note 13**). Concentration of the primary antibody should be reduced from 2- to 50-fold compared to the concentration used for conventional immunohistochemistry. We routinely use the anti-GFP antibody diluted between 1:1,000 and 1:2,000 (0.001–0.0005 mg/mL) in the conventional protocol. Using the TSA kit, the optimal concentration of anti-GFP was empirically determined to be between 1:4,000 and 1:10,000 (0.00025–0.0001 mg/mL).

8. Wash out primary antibody: three 5–10 min rinses with PBS.

9. HRP-conjugated secondary antibody: incubate sections for 2 h at room temperature (0.4–1 mL/well). The HRP-conjugated secondary goat anti rabbit antibody is diluted 1:100 (0.005 mg/mL) in the 1 % blocking reagent solution (*see* **Note 14**).

10. Wash out secondary antibody: three 5–10 min rinses with PBS.

11. Prepare TSA buffer: during final rinse in **step 10**, activate TSA buffer (Component E) with 0.0015 % of H_2O_2 (Component F) (*see* **Note 15**). Proceed in two steps to obtain a final concentration of 0.0015 % H_2O_2 using as little amplification buffer as possible. For example, for a volume of 1.2 mL, first add 1 μL of 30 % H_2O_2 solution to 19 μL of amplification buffer (dilution 1/20), then add 1.2 μL of this intermediate dilution to 1.2 mL of amplification buffer (dilution 1/1,000) to obtain a final dilution of 1/20,000 (from 30 to 0.0015 % H_2O_2).

12. Tyramide signal amplification: incubate sections in prepared tyramide working solution (0.4–1 mL/well) for 5–10 min at room temperature (*see* **Note 16**). Alexa Fluor-488-tyramide stock solution is diluted 1/100 in the activated TSA buffer. The tyramide working solution has to be prepared at the last moment to avoid early interaction between tyramides and H_2O_2 and kept protected from direct light to preserve fluorescent dyes.

13. Wash out TSA solution: three 5–10 min rinses with PBS.

14. Mount sections on slides: fill a large petri dish (5.5 in. diameter) with PBS and immerse slide and sections in it. Using the brush, gently position and fix the sections to the charged surface of a pre-labeled slide.

15. Dry slides: place in slide holder in a nearly vertical position for 10 min.

16. Rinse slides: briefly rinse slides with ddH_2O by submersion in a 50 mL conical Falcon tube. Dry for 10 min.

17. Coverslip: deposit Fluoromount-G mounting medium with DAPI (0.01 mg/mL) on the slides and apply coverslip. Add 0.5 μL of DAPI stock solution (20 mg/mL) to 1 mL of Fluoromount–G to obtain a final concentration of 0.01 mg/mL. This Fluoromount + DAPI solution can be stored at 4 °C protected from light for 2 weeks. The amount of mounting medium laid on the slide depends on the number of sections mounted per slide, but is typically 100–150 μL (*see* **Note 17**). Mounted slides are kept at 4 °C protected from light (*see* **Note 18**).

18. Image slides: image the immunolabeled sections using a fluorescent microscope. We used 10× (N.A: 0.45) objective of a Zeiss Axio Observer VivaTome Inverted Fluorescence Microscope (Waitt Advanced Biophotonics Center, Core Facility, Salk institute, San Diego, CA, USA), and 20× (N.A: 0.8) and 40× (water immersion, N.A: 1.2) objectives of a ZEISS Confocal LSM 780 (Waitt Advanced Biophotonics Center, Core Facility, Salk institute, San Diego, CA, USA) equipped with 405 and 488 nm laser lines. Use identical settings (e.g., exposure times, gain) for a given wavelength to compare immunostaining obtained with the TSA kit +/−no primary antibody control or a conventional immunostaining protocol (Fig. 3).

4 Notes

1. Sodium azide is useful for inhibiting microbial growth but inhibits HRP enzymatic activity. It must be removed from the sections by serial rinsing prior to TSA.

2. Other third party HRP-conjugated antibodies can be used in this step if, for example, the primary antibody was made in a species other than rabbit.

3. For free-floating brain sections, 30 μm thickness is a good compromise to avoid damage caused by handling of more delicate thinner sections and reduced antibody penetration in thicker sections. Aldehyde-fixed brain sections are preferred to fresh brain sections for TSA amplification. Indeed, PFA fixation

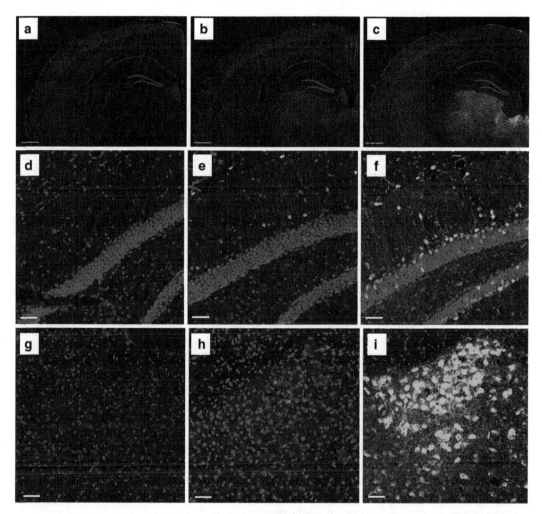

Fig. 3 Immunohistological comparison between conventional immunofluorescence and tyramide signal amplification. Coronal brain sections from a BAC-Tg VGLUT2-GFP mouse stained with anti-GFP antibodies to enhance signal. In the absence of immunolabel (**a, d, g**: no primary antibodies; control) little if any signal is detectable in aldehyde-fixed tissue. Conventional immunofluorescence using a Alexa Fluor-488-conjugated secondary antibody (**b, e, h**: *green*) reveals cell bodies, but only weak signal in subcellular processes. TSA enhancement (**c, f, i**: *green*) produces a more intense signal in the cell bodies and reveals additional subcellular processes. Sections were counterstained with DAPI (*blue*). (**a, b, c**) Wide-field image showing widespread GFP expression in subcortical thalamic structures but only weak and scattered expression in cortical and hippocampal structures (scale: 500 μm). Higher-magnification images taken through the (**d, e, f**) dentate gyrus of the hippocampus or (**g, h, i**) mediodorsal thalamic nucleus (scale: 50 μm)

generates protein cross-linking thus blocking endogenous peroxidase activity [23]. However, the fixative and fixation time can be critical variables and will depend on the tissue type and the primary antibody–epitope interaction. Protracted PFA fixation may generate free aldehyde groups in tissue resulting in a nonspecific labeling of conjugated antibodies [24].

4. TSA can be performed on slide-mounted sections or on free-floating sections. Immunolabeling performed directly on slides enables the use of smaller volumes of reagents compared to free-floating sections in plates. However, higher concentrations of antibody are often required due to less efficient antibody penetration, and nonspecific labeling around the borders of the tissue is a common occurrence.

5. Drying of sections may result in nonspecific labeling—antibodies may nonspecifically attach to dried tissue as a result of local ionic charges [24].

6. Gentle shaking of free floating sections during incubations improves tissue penetration and is essential to prevent layering and folding of the tissue on the bottom of the well. Agitation must be smooth to avoid tissue damage which makes mounting and imaging the samples more difficult.

7. Detergent permeabilizes cell membranes allowing antibodies to access and bind intra-cellular proteins.

8. Some cells or tissues contain endogenous peroxidases, for instance highly vascularized areas. The amplification reagent tyramide can interact with endogenous peroxidases generating nonspecific background signal. Pre-incubation with saturating amounts of H_2O_2 irreversibly blocks endogenous peroxidase activity and reduces background.

9. H_2O_2 is commonly used at 0.3, 1, and 3 %, typically for different durations, for example 30 min at 0.3 %, 20 min at 1 %, 5–10 min at 3 %. However, certain tissues, cells, or antigens (especially cell surface proteins) can be damaged by high concentrations of H_2O_2. We therefore recommend 0.3 % or 1 % for routine applications.

10. Triton X-100 (0.2 %) is typically included in the PBS rinses in conventional immunohistochemistry protocols.

11. In the conventional control immunostaining protocol using a fluorescent reporter-conjugated secondary antibody, the blocking solution is 4 % NDS diluted in PBS-T. Although not strictly necessary, serum blocking is generally more efficient (less background signal) if chosen from the same host species as the secondary antibody. For example, if the secondary antibody is donkey anti-rabbit, choose a normal donkey serum (NDS) to block nonspecific binding sites (e.g., Fc receptors, protein A, protein G). Normal serum can be replaced by 0.1–5 % bovine serum albumin (BSA). BSA containing blocking solution should also be made fresh prior to use.

12. For conventional immunostaining, primary antibodies were diluted in PBS-T and 4 % NDS. A very important no primary control was also performed and is highly recommended.

13. TSA for one epitope can be combined with conventional labeling for a second (and third) epitope using secondary antibodies conjugated to fluorophores with non-overlapping excitation/emission spectra. However, the species against which the secondary antibody is raised is a crucial concern. The HRP-conjugated anti-rabbit antibody in the TSA kit is cross-absorbed against human, mouse, and rat—thus cross reactivity with primary antibodies in other species may occur (for example, we have observed cross reactivity with sheep primary antibodies). Possible interactions must be tested prior to multi-labeling experiment using appropriate control conditions. For example, each primary antibody should be tested in isolation using multi-labeling conditions (i.e., with all secondary antibodies and other reagents included). We recommend including a no primary antibody control in all experiments.

14. In our parallel control experiment the HRP conjugate is replaced by a donkey anti-rabbit secondary antibody conjugated directly to Alexa Fluor-488 diluted at 1/400 (0.0025 mg/mL) in PBS-T.

15. Prepare H_2O_2 dilution at the last moment for maximal efficiency.

16. Prolonged exposure to H_2O_2 can increase background and reduce the fine subcellular resolution due to saturation of tyrosine residue binding sites and diffusion of activated tyramide away from the epitope.

17. For best results and to minimize bubbles, mounting medium can be laid in a horizontal line in the middle or edge of the slide or dispensed as drops on each of the sections. Practice this step on unstained or unneeded tissue sections.

18. Mounting medium will solidify over several days. For long-term storage of immunostained sections, slides can be kept at–20 °C.

References

1. Bobrow MN, Moen PT, Jr (2001) Tyramide signal amplification (TSA) systems for the enhancement of ISH signals in cytogenetics. Curr Protoc Cytom Chapter 8: Unit 8.9

2. Macechko PT, Krueger L, Hirsch B et al (1997) Comparison of immunologic amplification vs enzymatic deposition of fluorochrome-conjugated tyramide as detection systems for FISH. J Histochem Cytochem 45:359–363

3. Ormanns W, Schaffer R (1985) An alkaline-phosphatase staining method in avidin-biotin immunohistochemistry. Histochemistry 82: 421–424

4. Bobrow MN, Harris TD, Shaughnessy KJ et al (1989) Catalyzed reporter deposition, a novel method of signal amplification. Application to immunoassays. J Immunol Methods 125: 279–285

5. Bobrow MN, Shaughnessy KJ, Litt GJ (1991) Catalyzed reporter deposition, a novel method of signal amplification. II. Application to membrane immunoassays. J Immunol Methods 137: 103–112

6. Portsmann B, Portsmann T, Nugel E et al (1985) Which of the commonly used marker enzymes gives the best results in colorimetric

and fluorimetric enzyme immunoassays: horseradish peroxidase, alkaline phosphatase or beta-galactosidase? J Immunol Methods 79: 27–37

7. Zaidi AU, Enomoto H, Milbrandt J et al (2000) Dual fluorescent in situ hybridization and immunohistochemical detection with tyramide signal amplification. J Histochem Cytochem 48:1369–1375

8. Bobrow MN, Moen PT Jr (2001) Tyramide Signal Amplification (TSA) Systems for the Enhancement of ISH Signals in Cytogenetics. Current Protocols in Cytometry. Chapter 8:Unit 8.9

9. Mayer G, Bendayan M (1997) Biotinyl-tyramide: a novel approach for electron micro-scopic immunocytochemistry. J Histochem Cytochem 45:1449–1454

10. Van Heusden J, de Jong P, Ramaekers F et al (1997) Fluorescein-labeled tyramide strongly enhances the detection of low bromodeoxyuri-dine incorporation levels. J Histochem Cytochem 45:315–319

11. Raap AK, van de Corput MP, Vervenne RA et al (1995) Ultra-sensitive FISH using peroxidase-mediated deposition of biotin- or fluorochrome tyramides. Hum Mol Genet 4:529–534

12. van Gijlswijk RP, Wiegant J, Vervenne R et al (1996) Horseradish peroxidase-labeled oligo-nucleotides and fluorescent tyramides for rapid detection of chromosome-specific repeat sequences. Cytogenet Cell Genet 75:258–262

13. Sako W, Morigaki R, Kaji R et al (2011) Identification and localization of a neuron-specific isoform of TAF1 in rat brain: implica-tions for neuropathology of DYT3 dystonia. Neuroscience 189:100–107

14. Okita S, Morigaki R, Koizumi H et al (2012) Cell type-specific localization of optineurin in the striatal neurons of mice: implications for neuronal vulnerability in Huntington's disease. Neuroscience 202:363–370

15. Morigaki R, Sako W, Okita S et al (2011) Cyclin-dependent kinase 5 with phosphorylation of tyrosine 15 residue is enriched in striatal matrix

compartment in adult mice. Neuroscience 189: 25–31

16. Koizumi H, Morigaki R, Okita S et al (2013) Response of striosomal opioid signaling to dopamine depletion in 6-hydroxydopamine-lesioned rat model of Parkinson's disease: a potential compensatory role. Front Cell Neurosci 7:74

17. Zhao C, Eisinger B, Gammie SC (2013) Characterization of GABAergic neurons in the mouse lateral septum: a double fluorescence in situ hybridization and immunohistochemical study using tyramide signal amplification. PLoS One 8:e73750

18. van Gijlswijk RP, Zijlmans HJ, Wiegant J et al (1997) Fluorochrome-labeled tyramides: use in immunocytochemistry and fluorescence in situ hybridization. J Histochem Cytochem 45:375–382

19. Gong H, Byers DM (2003) Glutamate-41 of Vibrio harveyi acyl carrier protein is essential for fatty acid synthase but not acyl-ACP synthe-tase activity. Biochem Biophys Res Commun 302:35–40

20. Hnasko TS, Chuhma N, Zhang H et al (2010) Vesicular glutamate transport promotes dopa-mine storage and glutamate corelease in vivo. Neuron 65:643–656

21. Hnasko TS, Hjelmstad GO, Fields HL et al (2012) Ventral tegmental area glutamate neu-rons: electrophysiological properties and pro-jections. J Neurosci 32:15076–15085

22. Kapuscinski J (1990) Interactions of nucleic acids with fluorescent dyes: spectral properties of condensed complexes. J Histochem Cytochem 38:1323–1329

23. Horling L, Neuhuber WL, Raab M (2012) Pitfalls using tyramide signal amplification (TSA) in the mouse gastrointestinal tract: endogenous streptavidin-binding sites lead to false positive staining. J Neurosci Methods 204:124–132

24. Bussolati G, Leonardo E (2008) Technical pit-falls potentially affecting diagnoses in immuno-histochemistry. J Clin Pathol 61:1184–1192

Chapter 17

Correlative Microscopy for Localization of Proteins In Situ: Pre-embedding Immuno-Electron Microscopy Using FluoroNanogold, Gold Enhancement, and Low-Temperature Resin

Daniela Boassa

Abstract

Immuno-electron microscopy (immuno-EM) is a technique that has been used widely to determine sub-cellular localization of proteins. Different approaches are available for immuno-EM: pre-embedding method, post-embedding, and cryosectioning (Tokuyasu "style"). Here we describe a pre-embedding technique that allows the labeling of a target protein in situ, retention of fluorescence signal in plastic, and its localization at the EM level in a given cellular context. The procedure can be technically challenging and labor intensive: it requires optimization of fixation protocols to better preserve the cellular morphology and screening of compatible antibodies. Nevertheless, immuno-EM can be a powerful localization tool.

Key words Pre-embedding immuno-EM, FluoroNanogold, Gold enhancement, LR White, Normal rat kidney, Correlative microscopy, Fluorescence microscopy, Electron microscopy

1 Introduction

The main challenge in immuno-EM is the retention of antigenicity while preserving fine ultrastructure. The prerequisite to successful application of the method is the quality of the antibody in terms of good affinity and specificity for native proteins. Applicability of an antibody for western blot is not sufficient since this method detects denatured proteins. With immuno-EM the antibody has to recognize its epitope after aldehyde fixation and resin embedding which can remove up to 90 % of the epitopes. The first step in the method is to try the immunolabeling at the light microscopy level to test the antibody labeling under fixation conditions suitable for EM. Once the labeling obtained is satisfactory, the protocol can be adjusted to reach a compromise between preservation of ultrastructure and labeling. One of the advantages of pre-embedding

Robert Hnasko (ed.), *ELISA: Methods and Protocols*, Methods in Molecular Biology, vol. 1318, DOI 10.1007/978-1-4939-2742-5_17, © Springer Science+Business Media New York 2015

immuno-EM is that the labeling is done before the embedding, thereby avoiding the further loss of antigenicity during this step.

The development of FluoroNanogold (FNG) provided a marker system with a greater permeability and labeling sensitivity [1]. These probes comprise a 1.4 nm gold particle (Nanogold) conjugated to a Fab' fragment and a fluorescent label, allowing for imaging by correlative light and electron microscopy [2, 3]. Particularly, the combination of FNG with an intensification step (silver or gold intensification) enhanced the detection of intracellular antigens at the EM level by using pre-embedding methods.

The ability to track the distribution of macromolecular complexes by utilizing multiple imaging modalities is a valuable tool in biology and sparked a general interest over the years to develop various approaches for correlated/correlative microscopy. Current techniques include plastic embedding compatible with fluorescence preservation [4, 5]. Particularly, some hydrophilic resins are capable of low temperature polymerization, thereby avoiding denaturing proteins due to heat or stringent dehydration.

In this chapter we apply this method to visualize connexin43 proteins endogenously expressed in normal rat kidney (NRK) cells. With the use of LR White resin we were able to image the fluorescent signal from Cx43 proteins labeled with FNG in plastic, followed by the visualization of their subcellular localization by EM.

2   Materials

1. NRK cells plated on 35 mm glass-bottom dishes (MatTek Corporation, Ashland, MA) pre-coated with poly-d-lysine are grown in Dulbecco's modified Eagle's medium (Mediatech, Inc., Manassas, VA) supplemented with 10 % FBS in a humidified 5 % CO_2 incubator at 37 °C. Cells should be ~70–90 % confluent to be used for the experiment.

2. Buffered solutions. Hanks' Balanced Salt Solution (HBSS) with calcium and magnesium, no phenol red, 1×, pH 7.0 (Life Technologies). Phosphate-Buffered Saline (PBS), pH 7.0.

3. Antibodies. Primary antibody: rabbit polyclonal anti-Cx43 (dilution 1:400; Sigma, Cat. # C6219). Secondary antibodies: Alexa 488-FluoroNanogold goat anti-rabbit (dilution 1:100; Nanoprobes, Inc., Yaphank, NY) or FITC goat anti-rabbit (dilution 1:100; Jackson ImmunoResearch Laboratories, Inc., West Grove, PA).

4. Fixative. Prepare a 4 % (w/v) paraformaldehyde (PFA) solution in PBS. To make a volume of 50 ml: heat up 40 ml of ddH$_2$O at 60 °C with a stirring hot plate in a fume hood; turn off the hot plate and dissolve 2 g of PFA prills (Electron Microscopy Sciences) and while stirring add 25 μl of 5 N

NaOH. Filter the solution in a graduated cylinder using a filter paper. Add 5 ml of 10× PBS. Adjust pH to 7.4. Adding ddH$_2$O bring the volume to 50 ml.

4 % PFA/PBS + 0.1 % glutaraldehyde: add 200 µl of 25 % glutaraldehyde solution in 50 ml of freshly prepared PFA.

2 % PFA/PBS: follow same procedure as 4 % PFA/PBS adjusting the quantity of PFA prills according to the desired concentration.

2 % PFA/PBS + 0.1 % glutaraldehyde: add 200 µl of 25 % glutaraldehyde solution in 50 ml of freshly prepared PFA.

2 % glutaraldehyde/PBS: add 1 ml of 25 % glutaraldehyde solution in 11 ml PBS (1×), to obtain a total volume of 12 ml.

5. Quenching solution. 50 mM glycine in PBS. Dissolve 188 mg of glycine in 50 ml of PBS (1×).

6. Blocking/permeabilizing buffer. 1 % Bovine Serum Albumin (BSA), 5 % Normal Goat Serum (NGS), 0.1 % Triton X-100, 20 mM glycine, 1 % fish gelatin in PBS. Dissolve 0.5 g of BSA, 2.5 ml of NGS, 50 µl of Triton X-100, 0.075 g of glycine, and 500 µl of fish gelatin in 50 ml of PBS (1×).

7. Working buffer. Dilute blocking buffer 1:10 in PBS (1×).

8. Gold enhancement EM kit (Nanoprobes, Inc., Yaphank, NY). The mixture should be prepared just before use.

9. Ice-cold ethanol solutions: 20–50–70–90–100 %.

10. LR White resin (London Resin Company, Berkshire, England).

11. Aclar Embedding Film (Electron Microscopy Sciences).

12. 200 mesh copper grids (Electron Microscopy Sciences).

13. Diatome diamond knife for ultrathin sections (Electron Microscopy Sciences).

3 Methods

Perform a fixation series of paraformaldehyde and glutaraldehyde dilutions, and assess where the fluorescence signal is lost.

1. Remove the culture medium from the MatTek dishes containing the cells and wash three times with HBSS pre-warmed up at 37 °C. Fix cells with pre-warmed fixative at 37 °C (4 % PFA, 4 % PFA + 0.1 % glut, 2 % PFA, 2 % PFA + 0.1 % glut) for 5 min at room temperature followed by 30 min over ice. All solutions and steps from this point on are utilized and performed at 4 °C for the preservation of the ultrastructure (*see* **Note 1**).

2. Remove fixative and wash cells three times for 2 min each in ice-cold 1× PBS. Note: during any washing step the cells should never become dry to avoid irreversible damage to morphology.

3. Incubate in blocking buffer for 1 h at 4 °C (*see* **Note 2**).

4. Incubate in primary antibody diluted in *blocking buffer* at 4 °C for 1 h on a rocking platform set for gentle agitation (*see* **Note 3**).

5. Rinse cells with Working Buffer, six times for 2 min each at 4 °C.

6. Incubate in secondary antibody diluted in *blocking buffer* at 4 °C for 1 h on a gentle rocker, protected from light. *Remember:* keep cells in the *dark* from now on, to preserve fluorescence.

7. Rinse cells with Working Buffer, six times for 3 min each at 4 °C.

8. Wash cells with ice-cold 1× PBS, three times for 3 min each at 4 °C.

9. Check staining with a fluorescence microscope; proceed with EM processing *only* if good signal and specificity is observed. An example of the fluorescence immunolabeling for Cx43 in NRK cells is shown in Fig. 1.

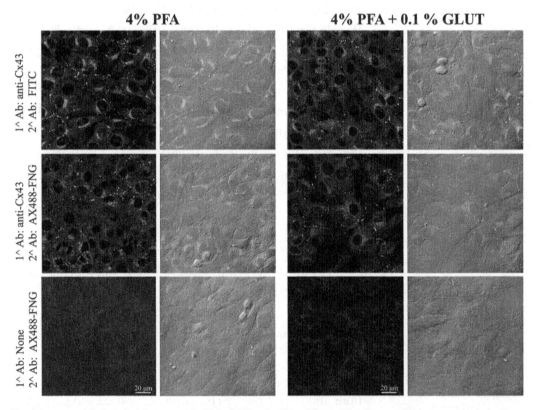

Fig. 1 Immunostaining of endogenous Cx43 in NRK cells. Two different fixative conditions were tested using a rabbit polyclonal anti-Cx43 antibody, a secondary goat anti rabbit Alexa Fluor 488-FluoroNanogold and a goat anti-rabbit FITC antibody. Gap junctions are clearly visible under all conditions tested, indicating the primary antibody tolerates the glutaraldehyde fixation. As control, primary antibody was omitted and no labeling was observed

10. Postfix with 2 % glutaraldehyde in PBS for 10 min at 4 °C.

11. Remove fixative and rinse three times for 2 min each in ice-cold 1× PBS. Then wash cells for 5 min in quenching solution at 4 °C to remove aldehydes (*see* **Note 4**).

12. Rinse three times for 5 min each in ddH$_2$O at 4 °C.

13. *Gold enhancement:* incubate cells in the Gold Enhancement kit for 1–5 min to intensify gold particles. The reaction is light insensitive so it can be carried out under normal room lighting. The kit is composed of 4 components: the enhancer (A), the activator (B), the initiator (C), and the buffer (D). Equilibrate the solutions at room temperature. Right before use, combine equal volumes of A and B first, wait 5 min then add equal amounts of C and D (*see* **Note 5**).

14. Thoroughly rinse three times for 5 min each in ddH$_2$O at 4 °C.

15. *Dehydration (ethanol series)*: dehydrate in increasing concentration of ethanol: 20, 50, 70, 90, and 2× 100 % ice-cold ethanol for 2 min each. Then rinse with 100 % ethanol at room temperature for 2 min.

16. *Infiltration and embedding*:

    • Remove 100 % ethanol and replace with a 50:50 mixture of low-temperature resin (LR White): ethanol 100 % for 20 min at room temperature.

    • Remove the mixture and replace with 100 % LR White for 1 h. MatTek dish can be stored overnight in unpolymerized resin at 4 °C.

    • The following day allow three more changes in 100 % of LR White within an hour.

17. *Cold-cure procedure*: In a glass vial add 10 ml of LR White and one drop of accelerator. Mix well but avoid introducing any air to the solution and immediately add to cells. Cover with a piece of Aclar Embedding film, avoiding any air bubbles. Place MatTek dish inside an aluminum dish with ethanol on ice to keep the temperature low. Keep it on ice until the resin polymerizes (30 min to an hour). Store at 4 °C.

At this point the cells can be imaged at the LM level: the signal of the fluorescent label is retained after the embedding procedure and the enhanced gold particles can be viewed by transmitted light. An example is shown in Fig. 2.

18. *Sectioning:* choose a region containing labeled cells and mount and trim the LR-White block. Cut ultrathin sections (70–90 nm) and collect them on EM copper grids. Dry grids on filter paper and store them in a grid case at room temperature. Examine the ultrathin sections by TEM (*see* Fig. 3).

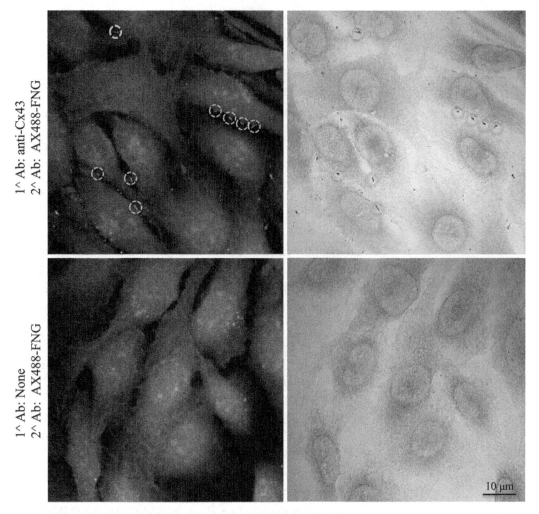

Fig. 2 Fluorescence preservation and gold labeling of endogenous Cx43 in NRK cells embedded in LR White resin. Following immunolabeling and gold intensification, cells embedded in LR White resin retained the Alexa Fluor 488 fluorescent signal (*green circles*, *left column*, *top row*). Transmitted light images (*right column*) show the corresponding gap junction puncta (*green circles*) visible as *darker spots* due to the gold intensification step. No labeling was observed in the control condition when the primary antibody was omitted (*bottom row*)

4 Notes

1. Fixatives are extremely hazardous and should be prepared and handled in a fume hood. Gloves and protective eyewear should be used at all times. PFA is a small fixative molecule and penetrates more rapidly into cells. Glutaraldehyde, though slower to penetrate, is a bifunctional crosslinker and therefore stabilizes the cellular components more efficiently. While PFA is typically used for light-level immunocytochemistry, allowing

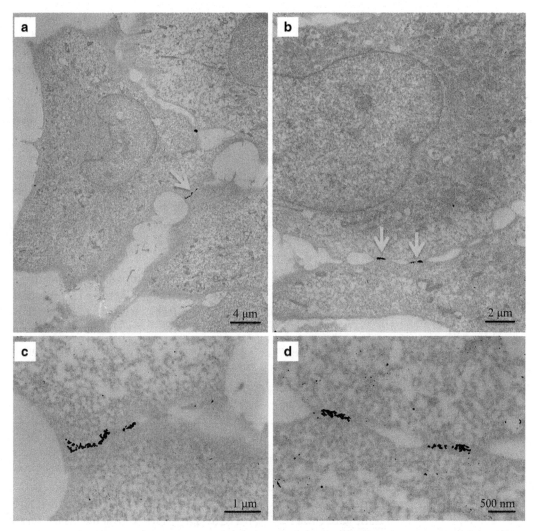

Fig. 3 Labeling of gap junctions after gold intensification. Electron micrographs showing gap junctions labeled by electron-dense gold particles (*green arrows* in **a** and **b**). Corresponding areas are shown at higher magnification in **c** and **d**

for overall antigen preservation, glutaraldehyde is a superior fixative for EM but can decrease the antigenicity significantly. For these reasons the ideal fixative for this method is a combination of the two to reach a balance between ultrastructure preservation and antigen retention.

2. For the localization of intracellular proteins such as Cx43, this protocol necessitates the use of a permeabilizing agent. In general, the use of detergents, although useful to facilitate the penetration of antibodies into cells, is detrimental for the preservation of the overall ultrastructure, which is why we recommend performing the permeabilization step at 4 °C.

For Triton X-100 we recommend not to exceed a concentration of 0.1 %. Several types of detergents are available and can be used as alternative to Triton X-100. For example, saponin is gentler with the membranes and is reversible and can be used to increase membrane permeabilization. Digitonin is another alternative. We recommend testing a series of dilutions with 0.1 % being the highest to assess the lowest concentration of detergent that will achieve a good labeling.

3. The optimal primary antibody dilution should be determined empirically for each antibody used. Also, the primary antibody incubation time can be different depending on the antibody used. Some might require a longer incubation time at 4 °C; others might work well only at room temperature. Whenever possible we recommend working at 4 °C in order to better preserve the ultrastructure.

4. The quenching step with glycine is important to inactivate unreacted aldehyde groups, which may be present after glutaraldehyde fixation. It does not affect negatively the ultrastructure preservation.

5. The size of the final gold particles depends of the time of application. Based on the target of interest the experimenter should adjust the time of gold enhancement.

Acknowledgement

We thank Tom Deerinck for expert technical advice. The work presented here was conducted at the National Center for Microscopy and Imaging Research at San Diego, which is supported by NIH Grant GM103412 awarded to Dr. Mark Ellisman. AHA Grant 10SDG2610281 (Daniela Boassa) supported this research.

References

1. Takizawa T, Robinson JM (2000) FluoroNanogold is a bifunctional immunoprobe for correlative fluorescence and electron microscopy. J Histochem Cytochem 48:481–485

2. Cheutin T, Sauvage C, Tchélidzé P, O'Donohue MF, Kaplan H, Beorchia A, Ploton D (2007) Visualizing macromolecules with FluoroNanogold: from photon microscopy to electron tomography. Methods Cell Biol 79:559–574

3. Hirano K, Kinoshita T, Uemura T, Motohashi H, Watanabe Y, Ebihara T, Nishiyama H, Sato M, Suga M, Maruyama Y, Tsuji NM, Yamamoto M, Nishihara S, Sato C (2014) Electron microscopy of primary cell cultures in solution and correlative optical microscopy using ASEM. Ultramicroscopy 143:52–66

4. Yang Z, Hu B, Zhang Y, Luo Q, Gong H (2013) Development of a plastic embedding method for large-volume and fluorescent-protein-expressing tissues. PLoS One 8(4): e60877

5. Watanabe S, Punge A, Hollopeter G, Willig KI, Hobson RJ, Davis MW, Hell SW, Jorgensen EM (2011) Protein localization in electron micrographs using fluorescence nanoscopy. Nat Methods 8(1):80–84

Chapter 18

Multiplex ELISA Using Oligonucleotide Tethered Antibodies

Robert S. Matson

Abstract

Multiplex assays represent a new paradigm for diagnostics. The simultaneous measure of multiple analytes from a single sample is advantageous in creating disease-associated panels that enable more accurate prognosis or diagnosis of the disease state. Furthermore, multiplexing may reduce reagent consumption, sample requirements and labor thereby lowering the cost per test. Here we describe a novel multiplex immunoassay technology based upon creating microarrays in microtiter plates that are formed upon the self-assembly of oligonucleotide–antibody conjugates.

Key words Multiplex, ELISA, Immunoassay, Oligonucleotide, Microarray, Self-assembly, Tethered, Interleukins, Cytokines, Oligo–antibody

1 Introduction

In this chapter we describe steps in preparing a quantitative multiplex immunoassay in a micro-plate format based upon the A^2 (A-squared) technology. Unlike conventional antibody microarrays in which antibodies are printed directly onto a substrate, the A^2 uses oligonucleotide tethering to attach antibodies to the surface. First, a polypropylene 96-well plate is surface treated for covalent attachment of capture oligonucleotides. Amine-terminated capture oligonucleotides are printed (*see* Fig. 1) in a 7×6 array pattern in each well of the plate (A^2 Plate).

Next, the complementary oligonucleotides are conjugated to selected antibodies to form the oligo–antibody conjugate (*see* Fig. 2).

The conjugates are pooled and added to the plate under hybridization conditions for the creation of the antibody array (*see* Fig. 3).

Once prepared, standard immunoassays may be conducted in multiplex [1].

What is the advantage of the A^2 approach? First, direct immobilization of antibodies often leads to random adsorption onto the surface and as pointed out by Cho et al., "random immobilization

Robert Hnasko (ed.), *ELISA: Methods and Protocols*, Methods in Molecular Biology, vol. 1318,
DOI 10.1007/978-1-4939-2742-5_18, © Springer Science+Business Media New York 2015

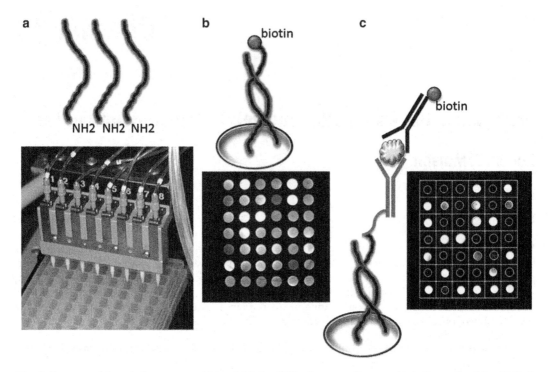

Fig. 1 Close-up of the printing process (**a**) in which the NH2-oligos are dispensed into the wells of the A2 Plate for covalent coupling in a 7 × 6 array format in each well. Complementary biotinylated oligos (**b**) are hybridized to the well and spots subsequently visualized by CCD camera detection (QuantiScientifics, A2 MicroArray System, cat. no. A21001) of fluorescent signal developed using a streptavidin-linked fluorescent conjugate. In image (**c**) the results of a multiplex sandwich ELISA are shown for a single well

results in a low rate (e.g., 5–10 %) of the active antibody density, that is, those that can participate in the binding reaction, which decreases even further when the substance to be analyzed is large in molecular size." [2]. Thus, stochastic conditions may result in reduced capture efficiency due to steric hindrance or potential blocking of the antibody binding site. Furthermore, printing of proteins can lead to significant variation in spot morphology and protein density thereby reducing array quality [3, 4]. Alternatively, the printing of well characterized capture oligonucleotides offers several advantages. First, oligonucleotide arrays are highly reproducible to produce and extremely stable. Oligonucleotide array plates when properly stored have a shelf-life extending beyond 5 years (QuantiScientifics). Because the formation of duplex DNA is thermodynamically controlled the density of the tethered oligo–antibody conjugates is relatively constant from spot to spot. As a result, the variation of immobilized antibody among spots is reduced which in turn aids in lowering assay imprecision.

The chapter is divided into three main methodologies: oligonucleotide–antibody conjugation, hybridization, and performing a multiplex immunoassay.

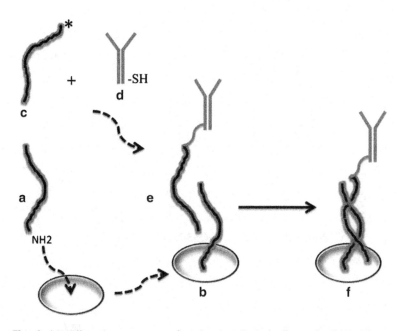

Fig. 2 14 different sequences of amine-terminated oligonucleotides (**a**) are printed in triplicate onto the well bottoms of an amine reactive polypropylene 96-well plate, the A² ®Plate, to form arrays of capture oligonucleotides (**b**). SMCC-activated complementary oligonucleotides (**c**) react with thiolated antibodies (**d**) to form oligo–antibody conjugates (**e**). The conjugates are pooled in a hybridization buffer and added to the wells of the capture oligo array plate to form a 42 spot antibody array in each well (**f**, single spot shown)

2 Materials

2.1 Components for Oligo–Antibody Conjugation

1. Solid Phase: butyl sepharose 4 fast flow (GE Healthcare), supplied as a slurry in ethanol (*see* **Note 1**). Store at 2–8 °C.

2. Initiator: iminothiolane (Sigma-Aldrich), hygroscopic and moisture sensitive (*see* **Note 2**). Store dry at 2–8 °C.

3. Binding Buffer: sodium phosphate, 20 mM containing sodium sulfate, 1 M, pH 7.5. Store at room temperature.

4. Elution Buffer: sodium phosphate, 20 mM, pH 7.5. Store at room temperature.

5. Spin-Columns: polypropylene centrifuge tube with attached cap, 0.8 mL internal volume (*see* **Note 3**), fritted disk (Sigma-Aldrich).

6. Activated Oligonucleotides: 4-(N-Maleimidomethyl) cyclohexane-1-carboxylic acid N-hydroxysuccinimidyl-terminated oligonucleotides (SMCC activated oligos, QuantiScientifics, cat. no. A21005), moisture sensitive. Store dry at –15 to –20 °C prior to use.

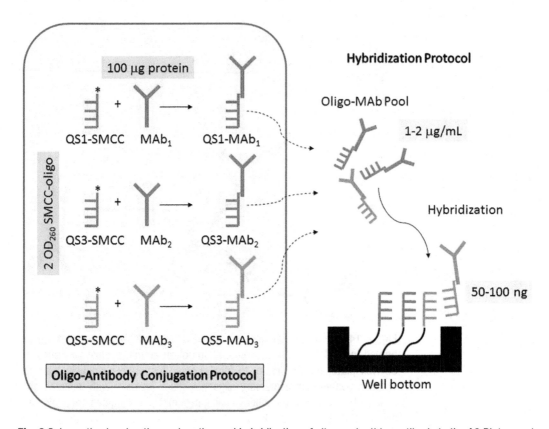

Fig. 3 Schematic showing the conjugation and hybridization of oligonucleotide–antibody to the A2 Plate creating a 3-plex antibody array in a well

Materials and Equipment

Micro Centrifuge: $400 \times g$.

Rotator: end-over-end type or nutating mixer.

Pipettors: single channel.

Pipet Tips: 100–1,000 μL capacity.

Glass pipet: 5 mL.

UV/VIS Spectrophotometer.

Cuvettes.

Micro BCA Protein Assay Kit (Thermo Scientific, cat. no. 23235).

Capture Antibody: 100 μg, purified at a concentration of ≥ 1 mg/mL (*see* **Note 4**). Storage buffer must be free of reactive thiols.

2.2 Components for Oligo–Antibody Conjugate Hybridization to Capture Oligo Plate

Hybridization Buffer A (QuantiScientifics, cat. no. A21003-HYB A): contains formamide (*see* **Note 5**); avoid contact. Follow proper laboratory safety procedures for handling and storage. Store at 2–8 °C.

Hybridization Buffer B (QuantiScientifics, cat. no A21003-HYB B): supplied for direct use. Store at 2–8 °C.

Biotinylated Reference Oligo (QuantiScientifics, cat. no. A21003-REF): supplied ready for use. Store at 2–8 °C.

Wash Buffer: tris buffered saline with Tween 20, pH 8.0 (TBST, Sigma-Aldrich), 0.05 M Tris–HCl, 0.138 M NaCl, 0.0027 M KCl, Tween 20, 0.05 %. Store at room temperature.

Materials and Equipment

A2 Plate (QuantiScientifics, cat. no. A21002).

Polypropylene Centrifuge Tube, 15 mL, conical.

Platform Shaker (gyratory).

Pipettors: single channel and multichannel.

Pipet Tips: 0–200 μL capacity.

2.3 Components for Performing the Multiplex ELISA

Reagents

Streptavidin Alkaline Phosphatase (Thermo Scientific): dilute 1:20,000 (v/v) in TBST to prepare a working stock solution (*see* **Note 6**).

Streptavidin SureLight P-1 (Columbia BioSciences): dissolve 150 μg solid with 150 μL distilled water to prepare 50× primary stock concentrate. Dilute stock 1:50 (v/v) in TBST just prior to use as a working stock solution.

Materials and Equipment

A2 Capture Antibody Array Plate: previously prepared.

Platform Shaker (gyratory).

Pipettors: single channel or multichannel.

Pipet tips: 0–200 μL capacity.

A2 MicroArray Reader (QuantiScientifics, cat. no. A21001): Optical Cube A installed, Ex 545 nm, Em 650 nm and/or Optical Cube B installed, Ex 480 nm, Em 535 nm (*see* **Note 7**).

3 Methods

3.1 Conjugations

This protocol is for the preparation of oligonucleotide–antibody conjugates for use with the A^2 ® Plate Array. Approximately 2 $OD_{260\ nm}$ units of an activated oligonucleotide are reacted with 100 μg of purified antibody (IgG). The process involves adsorption of the immunoglobulin onto a solid-phase held within a chromatographic column (or large spin-column). Next, initiator is added to modify the antibody with reactive sulfhydryl (-SH) groups. Finally, the SMCC-oligonucleotide is added which couples

Table 1
Expected yield of the oligonucleotide–antibody conjugate using IgG from different animal species

Species	Yields
Mouse (pAb and mAb)	40–70 %
Goat	65–80 %
Rabbit	60–70 %
Guinea pig	30–50 %

to the thiolated antibody to form the oligo–antibody conjugate. The resulting conjugate still bound to the solid-support is rinsed free of reactants; and subsequently eluted in purified form from the column ready for use. Conjugation yield varies with the IgG species (*see* Table 1).

Protocol

Solid-Phase: bring to room temperature prior to use; gently mix slurry to dispense.

Spin Column: place bottom cap on column tip and insert capped spin column into a collection tube.

Prepare Spin Columns

1. Add 100 µL of a well-mixed solid-phase slurry to spin column (*see* **Note 8**).

2. Spin: 2,000 rpm, 30 s.

3. Discard solution.

4. Add 600 µL DDI H_2O and mix bed by up and down with a pipette.

5. Spin and discard rinse.

6. Repeat **steps #4, #5**.

7. Add 600 µL binding buffer and mix bed by up and down with a pipette.

8. Spin and discard rinse.

9. Repeat **steps #7, #8**.

10. Cap bottom of spin column.

11. Cap top until ready for use.

Prepare Antibody Binding

1. Remove top cap from spin column.

2. Add 100 µL antibody solution directly to the bed and mix with pipette (*see* **Note 9**).

3. Add 500 µL binding buffer to the column bed.

4. Mix bed by up and down by pipette action.

5. Securely cap top of the column.

6. Tumble: 10 min.

7. Remove bottom cap and spin 2,000 rpm, 30 s.

8. Measure OD_{280} in effluent: if OD280 > 0.01 reapply effluent and repeat tumble.

9. If OD_{280} < 0.01 then cap bottom of spin column, ready for next steps.

Prepare Protein Initiator

1. Weigh out ~1.9 mg initiator (*see* **Note 10**).

2. Dissolve in 1 mL binding buffer.

3. For one spin column: combine 50 µL (**step #2**) with 750 µL binding buffer.

4. Add the entire volume from **step #3** (800 µL) to the spin column and mix bed by pipetting.

5. Cap top and seal with Parafilm (*see* **Note 11**).

6. Tumble: 1 h at room temperature.

7. Remove bottom cap (change collection tube).

8. Wash with 600 µL binding buffer.

9. Spin and discard rinse.

10. Repeat **steps #8, #9**- five (5) more times.

11. Cap bottom of spin column, ready for next steps.

Prepare Activated Oligo

1. Spin down tube containing activated oligo (2 OD_{260}) to pellet contents.

2. Reconstitute activated oligo in 800 µL binding buffer, mix well and spin tube again.

3. Add oligo solution to the spin column.

4. Mix column bed by up and down pipetting action.

5. Replace top cap and seal with Parafilm.

6. Tumble: overnight (15–20 h) at room temperature.

Prepare Oligo–Antibody Conjugate

1. Remove caps and spin 2,000 rpm, 30 s.

2. Replace collection tube to collect washes.

3. Wash with 600 µL binding buffer and check OD_{260}.

4. Repeat washes until OD_{260} < 0.01.

5. Discard washes.

6. Change collection tubes.

7. Add 100 μL of elution buffer and mix well by pipetting action.

8. Spin: 2,000 rpm, 30 s.

9. Recover the eluate into a labeled 1 mL collection tube.

10. Repeat four more times with 100 μL elutions (500 μL total) collected into the same collection tube used in **step #9** (*see* **Note 12**).

11. Determine protein content of the collected eluate using the BCA method.

12. Store conjugates at 2–8 °C in preparation for hybridization to the A2 Plate.

3.2 Hybridization

This protocol is for the creation of the A2 Capture Antibody Array by hybridization of the previously prepared Oligonucleotide–Antibody Conjugates. The conjugates are pooled into a hybridization cocktail prepared by mixing Hybridization Buffers A and B; and then applied to the A2 Plate. The number of plates that can be prepared depends upon the conjugate yield and desired loading (*see* Table 2).

Protocol

1. Combine 6 μg of each of the conjugates together in a 15 mL centrifuge tube (*see* **Note 13**).

2. Add 18 μL of the biotinylated reference oligonucleotide to the tube.

Table 2
Determining the number of potential A2 oligo–antibody plates based upon conjugate yield and loading

	Conjugation yield (total μg available/100 μg coupling)									
	100	90	80	70	60	50	40	30	20	10
	# Oligo–antibody plates:									
0.3 Plate Loading (μg/mL)	63	57	51	44	38	32	25	19	13	6
0.5	38	34	30	27	23	19	15	11	8	4
1	19	17	15	13	11	9	8	6	4	2
1.5	13	11	10	9	8	6	5	4	3	1
2	9	9	8	7	6	5	4	3	2	1
2.5	8	7	6	5	5	4	3	2	2	1
3	6	6	5	4	4	3	3	2	1	1

Number of A^2 plates prepared with oligo–antibody conjugate

3. Add 1,500 µL HYB Buffer A.

4. Add HYB Buffer B to reach a final total volume of 6,000 µL.

5. Mix well.

Hybridization

1. Bring the A2 Plate to room temperature prior to removing from its pouch (*see* **Note 14**).

2. Add 200 µL of Wash Buffer (1×) to each well of the A2 Plate.

3. Soak 5 min with shaking.

4. Remove the wash buffer but do not allow the plate to dry.

5. Tap the plate upside down onto several layers of clean towels to remove residual buffer.

6. Deliver 55 µL of the oligo–antibody pool to each well of the 96-well A2 Plate.

7. Cover the plate with a lid.

8. Incubate for 1 h at room temperature with shaking (100–300 rpm).

9. Remove the hybridization solution from the wells and discard.

10. Add 200 µL of Wash Buffer (1×) to each well and shake for 1 min.

11. Remove the wash buffer quickly by inverting over a sink.

12. Tap the plate upside down onto several layers of clean towels to remove residual buffer.

13. Repeat the wash (**steps #10–12**) an additional 2 times.

14. Place the lid back onto the plate.

15. Return the plate to the aluminum pouch containing the drying packet and seal.

16. Store the plate at 2–8 °C until need for the assay.

3.3 Multiplex ELISA

This protocol is for the performance of an Enzyme Linked Immunosorbent Assay (ELISA), using A² ® Plate with immobilized oligo–antibody array. The previously prepared oligo–antibody conjugates are pooled and applied to the A2 Plate (A21002) under hybridization conditions, resulting in the self-assembly of a capture antibody array in each well of the 96-well plate. After rinsing, the plate is ready to perform the multiplex ELISA. An example of a quantitative multiplex ELISA using this protocol is provided (*see* Fig. 4 and Table 3).

1. Bring the A2 Plate to room temperature prior to removing from its pouch.

2. Rehydrate by delivering 200 µL of Wash Buffer (1×) to each well of the A2 Plate.

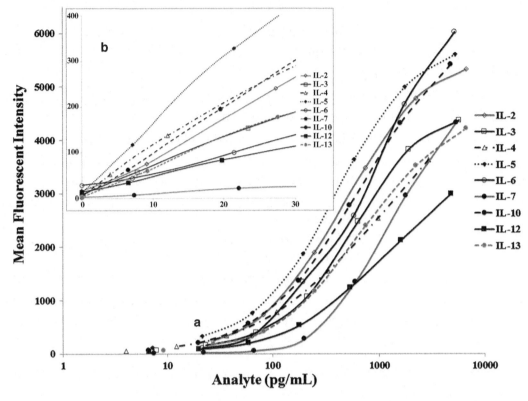

Fig. 4 9-plex Cytokine A2 Multiplex ELISA showing dynamic range in log scale (**a**) from 1 to 10,000 pg/mL of the interleukin (cytokine) analytes; and insert (**b**) linear range at lower limit of detection from 0 to 30 pg/mL

3. Soak for 5 min with shaking (250–300 rpm).

4. Remove the wash buffer but do not allow the plate to dry (*see* **Note 15**).

5. Tap the plate upside down onto several layers of clean towels to remove residual buffer.

6. Deliver 55 μL of previously prepared standards or sample to each well in appropriate diluents.

7. Incubate for 1 h at room temperature with shaking.

8. Remove solution as previously described.

9. Rinse wells 3 times with 200 μL Wash Buffer (1×) with a 5-min soak between rinses.

10. Deliver 55 μL of biotinylated antibody (in biotin antibody diluent) to each well.

11. Incubate for 1 h at room temperature with shaking.

12. Remove solution and rinse wells 3 times with 200 μL Wash Buffer (1×) with 5-min soaks.

Table 3
A2 MicroArray System report for multiplex ELISA results. The values represent duplicate assays evaluated using a 4-Parameter Logistic (4 PL) regression plot

IFN-g						
Net Avg Int	Std dev	%CV	Obs conc	Exp conc	% Recovery	Serial dilution
4,368	208	4.8	1,992.2	2,000.0	100	Undiluted
3,194	164	5.1	671.5	666.7	101	1/3
1,674	54	3.2	219.1	222.2	99	1/9
693	30	4.4	76.5	74.1	103	1/27
225	10	4.5	23.9	24.7	97	1/81
75	4	6.0	7.8	8.2	94	1/243
31	3	9.9	2.8	2.7	101	1/729
11	7	61.4	0.2	0.0		Blank
23.6						Blank +2SD

Gmcsf						
Net avg int	Std dev	%CV	Obs conc	Exp conc	% Recovery	Serial dilution
5,327	262	4.9	6,218.3	5,680.0	109	Undiluted
4,511	313	6.9	1,720.4	1,893.3	91	1/3
3,492	185	5.3	665.6	631.1	105	1/9
2,051	149	7.3	208.1	210.4	99	1/27
999	66	6.6	68.7	70.1	98	1/81
437	34	7.9	23.5	23.4	100	1/243
169	11	6.2	7.5	7.8	97	1/729
9	6	68.6	0.3	0.0		Blank
21.6						Blank +2SD

IL-10						
Net avg int	Std dev	%CV	Obs conc	Exp conc	% Recovery	Serial dilution
5,408	411	7.6	4,792.8	4,750.0	101	Undiluted
4,307	328	7.6	1,565.1	1,583.3	99	1/3
2,775	160	5.8	532.2	527.8	101	1/9
1,366	89	6.5	175.9	175.9	100	1/27
557	15	2.7	58.4	58.6	100	1/81
195	10	5.3	18.6	19.5	95	1/243
63	2	3.7	6.0	6.5	91	1/729
6	5	92.1	1.1	0.0		Blank
16.9						Blank +2SD

13. Deliver 55 µL of streptavidin-AP (1:20,000 v/v) to each well

14. Incubate for 30 min at room temperature with shaking.

15. Remove solution and rinse wells 3 times with 200 µL Wash Buffer (1×) with 5-min soaks.

16. Deliver 55 µL of AP Enzyme Substrate to each well.

17. Cover plate with foil or place in dark.

18. Incubate for 30 min at room temperature *without* shaking (*see* **Note 16**).

19. Carefully remove most of the solution from wells, *but* do not rinse or allow plate wells to dry out.

20. Wipe off the bottom of the plate with ethanol using a scratch free and lint free cloth.

21. Read the semi-wet plate on the A2 Reader (Channel **B**; 200 ms).

3.4 Multiplex Fluorescent Immunoassay

This protocol is similar to that described in Subheading 3.3 for Multiplex ELISA, except streptavidin alkaline phosphatase signal amplification is replaced by a streptavidin dye reporter (Columbia Biosciences, Streptavidin SureLight P-1).

1. Perform assay **steps #1–12**, as previously described in Subheading 3.3.

2. Deliver 55 μL of a working stock solution of streptavidin P-1 to each well.

3. Incubate for 1 h at room temperature with shaking.

4. Remove solution and rinse wells 3 times with 200 μL Wash Buffer (1×) with 5-min soaks between rinses.

5. Fill wells with 200 μL of fresh Wash Buffer.

6. Wipe off the bottom of the plate with ethanol using a scratch free and lint free cloth.

7. Read the plate on the A2 Reader (Channel **A**; 200 ms).

4   Notes

1. In order to adsorb 100 μg of protein a packed gel bed of about 0.1 mL must be used in the spin column. Since the percentage of solids in the slurry may verify from lot to lot, the packed bed volume should be determined in advance. Use a spin column or graduated microcentrifuge tube to measure the required volume of slurry to achieve a 0.1 mL packed bed volume.

2. It is advisable to pre-weigh the iminothiolane (initiator) into several glass screw-cap vials; and then store sealed with drying agent in the refrigerator. First, bring the iminothiolane bottle to room temperature. Using a clean, dry spatula dispense into the glass vial. If possible, use amber glass vials (7 mL). Target a weigh out of about 2–3 mg (0.0020–0.0030 g). Calculate the initiator weight = Wt (vial + initiator)–Wt (vial), to the nearest 0.1 mg (±0.0001 g).

3. Use polypropylene spin columns with graduations to estimate the packed bed volume. Either compression style caps or screw

cap spin columns may be used. A column volume of 0.8–1.0 mL is required for this protocol.

4. The protocol requires that the binding capacity of the gel should be at least 100 µg antibody per 100 µL of packed bed. In order to achieve optimal adsorption, a protein concentration of at least 1 mg/mL is recommended. Addition of 100 µg of a more dilute antibody solution significantly alters the ionic strength of the buffer thereby reducing binding of the antibody to the matrix. Therefore, it is recommended that dilute antibody be concentrated in PBS to at least 1 mg/mL using a MWCO spin filter or other ultrafiltration concentrator. For example, Pierce Protein Concentrator, PES 10,000 MWCO spin filter (Thermo Scientifics, cat. no. 88513).

5. Hybridization of the oligo–antibody conjugate is accomplished using a formamide based hybridization cocktail that normalizes the T_m's for the pooled conjugates. A final formamide concentration of ~ 20–25 % (v/v) must be maintained. Thus, for a full plate, 6,000 µL of the Hyb Cocktail is prepared with 1,500 µL Hyb A buffer (formamide) and a combined volume of 4,500 µL = Hyb B buffer + Oligo–Ab Pool + Reference Oligo. Alternatively, a Hyb Cocktail can be premixed containing the reference oligonucleotide and stored under refrigeration for later use. Pooled oligo–antibody conjugates can then be added as required in a total volume (pool) not to exceed 20 % of the final volume (pool + Hyb Cocktail), e.g., 10 µL of 10 conjugates (100 µL pool) is combined with 500 µL Hyb Cocktail = 500 (25 %)/600 = 20.8 % formamide.

6. The enzymatic activity for streptavidin alkaline phosphatase will vary from lot to lot and vendor to vendor product. It is advisable to titer the enzyme to avoid any Hook Effect that may occur at higher enzyme concentrations. We have found that 1:10,000–1:20,000 dilution of enzyme is often required.

7. The A2 MicoArray System uses Axio Optical Cubes (Zeiss) consisting of excitation, dichroic and emission filters in the housing. Filter pairs and assembles are also available from several vendors including Chroma (Bellows Falls, VT) and Semrock, Inc (Rochester, NY).

8. The slurry tends to rapidly settle out. Make sure that the slurry is uniformly mixed, then immediately withdraw the required volume with a pipette and dispense into the spin column. Do not use a magnetic stirrer to disperse the slurry since this action may damage the beads. We have found that a shaker on high speed works well for such purpose.

9. The antibody solution is delivered directly to the packed bed pre-equilibrated in binding buffer in order to achieve maximal binding. No more than 100 µL of protein solution should

be applied, however, delivery of smaller volumes of more concentrated antibody solution are acceptable.

10. If possible the initiator solution should be adjusted to 1.9 mg/mL in binding buffer. Pre-weighed vials will permit calculation of the required volume of binding buffer to prepare. For example, 1 mg initiator may be dissolved in 526 μL of buffer, i.e., $1/1.9 = 0.526$

11. On occasion we have found that capped spin columns will leak. To prevent leakage from happening tightly wrap the column cap and top of the barrel with Parafilm.

12. Alternatively, elute may be collected stepwise in five separate fractions of 100 μL and protein determined for each fraction. Usually, the bulk of the conjugate elutes in the first three fractions and tails into fractions four and five. Thus, a more concentrated oligo–antibody conjugate can be obtained if desired.

13. Approximately 6 μg (6,000 μL total volume) of each oligo–antibody conjugate is consumed per 96-wells of the A2 Plate. This is based upon achieving delivery of each at 1 μg/mL per well: 55 μL/well × 96 wells = 5,280 μL × 1.136 = 6,000 μL. The amount of conjugate maybe varied to achieve optimal hybridization, usually between 0.3 and 3 μg/mL input concentration.

14. The A2 Plate should be rehydrated prior to use to achieve uniform wetting during hybridization.

15. Be careful not to touch the well bottom with the pipette tip in order to avoid damage to the array.

16. Alkaline Phosphatase catalyzes the formation of a fluorescent precipitate that is localized on the spots. Excessive mixing may results in partial dissolution of the precipitate into the bulk solution where it may redeposit elsewhere leading to an increase in the background fluorescence.

17. Long Term Storage of Conjugates: for storage beyond 3 months, it is recommended that the oligo–antibody conjugates be diluted 1:2 (v/v) with glycerol and stored at–20 °C.

18. For serum-based assays antigen standards should be prepared in solutions closely matching that of the sample matrix. For work with serum samples, dilute standards and samples (1:2 v/v or greater) in a diluent containing fetal calf serum.

19. Biotinylated Antibodies: pool the required secondary antibodies in diluent containing 1 % BSA. Deliver to the well at a final concentration for *each* at ~0.5 to~3 μg/mL. It is recommended that the optimal concentration for each secondary antibody be individually determined prior to pooling to achieve the best results.

References

1. Robbins MA, Li M, Leung I, Li H, Boyer DV, Song Y, Behlke M, Rossi JJ (2006) Stable expression of shRNAs in human CD34+ progenitor cells can avoid induction of interferon responses to siRNAs in vitro. Nat Biotechnol 24(5):566–571

2. Cho I-H, Seo S-M, Jeon J-W, Se-Hwan Paek S-H (2009) Characterization for binding complex formation with site-directly immobilized antibodies enhancing detection capability of cardiac troponin I. J Biomed Biotechnol 2009:104094. doi:10.1155/2009/10409

3. Montagu J (2009) Investigating assay precision and validation on different multiplex immunoassay platforms. Decision Biomarkers, New York

4. Bastarche JA, Koyama T, Wickersham NE, Mitchell DB, Mernaugh RL, Ware LB (2011) Accuracy and reproducibility of a multiplex immunoassay platform: a validation study. J Immunol Methods 367(1–2):33–39

Chapter 19

Gas Plasma Surface Chemistry for Biological Assays

Khoren Sahagian and Mikki Larner

Abstract

Biological systems respond to and interact with surfaces. Gas plasma provides a scalable surface treatment method for designing interactive surfaces. There are many commercial examples of plasma-modified products. These include well plates, filtration membranes, dispensing tools, and medical devices. This chapter presents an overview of gas plasma technology and provides a guide to using gas plasma for modifying surfaces for research or product development.

Keywords Plasma, Surface treatment, Functionalization, Immobilization, Conjugation, Hydrophobic, Hydrophilic, Gas plasma, Vacuum plasma, Amine, Carboxyl, Hydroxyl

1 Introduction

Gas plasma processes are utilized on a variety of materials for the purpose of engineering a working surface. A well-structured surface chemistry enables attachment of many biologically relevant molecules such as: antibodies, antigens, proteins, gels, and other macromolecules. The plasma based surface modification may be performed on a wide range of materials from metals to glass to polymers.

Plasma surface modification of polymers is a growing field. It is important to note that many of the first plasma systems entered into service for the purpose of surface etching. Surface etching generally refers to a method of removing or cutting into a surface. Such plasma technologies found wide adoption within the semiconductor industry for their nanoscale precision and uniformity. However these plasma etching tools were not especially suited for addition of surface chemistry on three-dimensional (3D) and thermally sensitive materials such as polymers. Thus the development of equipment configurations to allow for treatment of materials in a variety of forms from powders to extruded tubing to large rolls (*see* Figs. 1, 2).

Robert Hnasko (ed.), *ELISA: Methods and Protocols*, Methods in Molecular Biology, vol. 1318,
DOI 10.1007/978-1-4939-2742-5_19, © Springer Science+Business Media New York 2015

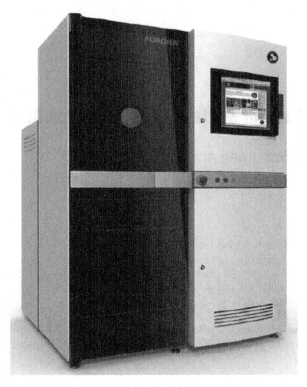

Fig. 1 Example Plasma Reactor System, manufactured by Plasmatreat

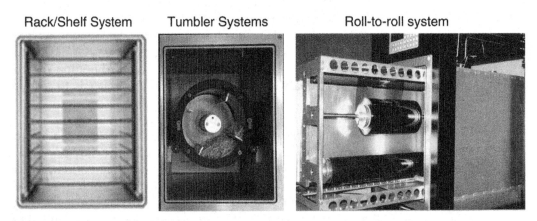

Fig. 2 Plasma system chamber configurations. Shown from *left to right*, Plasmatreat Aurora 350, Plasma Science 0500 Tumbler, Plasma Science 524 roll-to-roll system

These equipment and process advances have contributed to commercially scalable and reproducible stable surface modifications. Gas plasma technologies are increasingly innovating surface engineering through automation and process efficiencies.

Charged particles and disassociated chemical bonds make up gas plasma. These particles may become ionized with heat or a strong electromagnetic field. Sufficient energy must be applied to a system in order to produce plasma. The plasma may be generated under atmospheric pressure or under partial vacuum pressure. A few distinct advantages of an atmospheric plasma system are in-line processing, rapid treatment speeds, and compact line-of-sight automation. A system for producing plasma under partial vacuum pressure typically involves batch treatment within a vessel; however continuous treatments of transported profiles do exist. The distinct advantages of partial vacuum plasma are 3D surface treatments, environmental control, chemical versatility, and the modification of porous structure. Notably, a partial vacuum process also enables lower temperature plasma. Such plasma systems are able to produce tailored surface chemistry onto thermally sensitive materials. Additionally these methods provide atomic-level cleaning, stable surface wetting and deposition of thin organic films.

Plasma treatment technologies modify surfaces without affecting the bulk material properties (*see* **Note 1**). These methods provide inexpensive and controlled alternatives to custom material formulation and to traditional wet chemistry processing. In many cases low cost or commodity lab ware surfaces may be reengineered into high-performance substrates for cell culture, selective filtration, and discovery.

Partial pressure plasma reactors offer the user a versatile tool for creating tailored working surfaces. Tools for design include the equipment, chemistry and control of the variables described herein. Since practiced in a controlled reduced pressure environment, once a process has been validated, and materials specified, the operator can expect reproducibility. While plasma processing has grown into a distinct field of practice, the user can evaluate and prepare research and production tools simply by evaluation of and consideration of the variables discussed in this chapter.

2   Materials and Equipment Configuration

A list of materials that are commercially plasma-modified for biological assays are provided in Table 1. Bulk properties often make up the initial criteria for material selection (*see* **Note 1**). Examples include optical transmission, material processability, cost, biocompatibility, and gas or vapor transmission. When the surface does not meet performance requirements such as stable wetting or surface polarity for compatibility with biological fluids and reagents, gas plasma is a manufacturing solution for molecular reengineering of the surface to enable hydrophilicity, hydrophobicity, and linkers for covalent bonding for example. These linkers may be designed to be closely coupled or spaced, enabling tailoring for maximum attachment of the molecule without steric hindrance.

Table 1
Materials used in biological assay development

Material	Product form	Plasma process
Cyclo-olefin polymer or copolymer	Microtiter plate	Stable wetting, functional surfaces
Polystyrene	Microtiter plate, pipettes	Stable wetting, functional surfaces
Polycarbonates	Microtiter plate	Stable wetting, functional surfaces
Glass (borosilicate, quartz)	Pipettes	Functional surfaces
Fluoropolymers	Dispensing components, transfer membranes	Stable wetting
Polypropylene	Pipettes	Stable wetting
PEEK	Dispensing components	
Sintered polyethylene	Wicks, capillaries, filtration, transfer membranes	Hydrophilicity, hydrophobicity, enhance binding, enhance flow
Nitrocellulose	Wicks, capillaries, filtration, transfer membranes	Hydrophobic
Stainless steel	Dispensing components	Stable wetting, hydrophobic, air bubble mitigation, low retention coatings, wear resistance

There are many components considered common to systems which produce plasma under partial vacuum pressure. The equipment used for the processes described in this chapter was manufactured by Plasma Science, Plasma Technology Systems and Plasmatreat. Equipment configurations are selected upon the throughput requirements and product form factor (*see* Fig. 2). The following is a list of common components in equipment used by the authors [1].

Reaction Chamber: The portion of the system which generates the plasma. The chamber volume is sealed from atmosphere (*see* **Note 8**). Parts are loading into the chamber on trays or with a custom fixture (*see* **Note 5**). The trays may be electrically isolated, powered, or ground.

Process Controller: The Process Controller is the module that monitors all the sensors and transducers, stores the program into nonvolatile memory, displays pertinent data, and assures program execution.

HMI: The Plasma HMI (Human Machine Interface) is the primary display and peripheral hardware for monitoring the Process Controller and for initiating instruction. It allows the user to recall programmed recipes, to commence a process in manual or automatic modes, to edit set points, to enable manually activated devices, to view trends, to view alarms, and to export data for analysis to comply with FDA Part 21CFR 11 electronic record requirements.

RF Generator: A module whose function is to generate high-frequency radio frequency (RF) power. Equipment used by the authors is configured with 13.56 MHz, solid state generators. The RF power from the generator provides the energy required to create plasma.

Matching Network: A module whose function is to assure efficient transfer of RF energy from the RF Generator into the Reaction Chamber electrodes. With proper matching, plasma is reproducibly maintained regardless of the chamber load and/or changes in pressure (*see* **Note 3**.)

Electrodes: The electrodes, which are located in the reaction chamber, conduct the energy from the generator. It is this energy that creates the plasma. Electrode configurations vary, with capacitively coupled (two electrodes separated by a small distance) as the primary arrangement for the equipment used by the authors. An illustration of this arrangement is shown in Fig. 3.

Gas/Vapor Flow Controllers: Mass Flow Controllers (MFC) or Liquid Flow Controllers (LFC) is a feedback control device

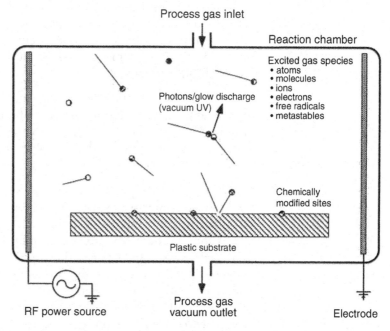

Fig. 3 Schematic of surface modification in a gas plasma reactor

designed to regulate gas or vapor flow rates to a desired set point. The MFC/LFC reproduces flow rate independent of temperature and inlet or outlet pressure (*see* **Note 3**.)

Pressure Transducer: The transducer, also known as a capacitance manometer, is a sensor for measuring chamber pressure under partial vacuum. The output signal is read by the plasma Process Controller (*see* **Note 3**.)

Vacuum pump: The pump is plumbed to the Reaction Chamber by vacuum conduit. The function of the Vacuum Pump is to reduce the chamber to operating pressure, and to expel used process gases. Pump selection is important for achieving adequate pumping capacity. Outgassing such that occurs with polymers and materials with high moisture uptake (where the moisture is not favorable for processing) requires high pumping capacity. Outgassed species are removed by the pump so that they do not become products in the plasma. Pump configurations vary and should be selected to ensure compatibility with the process chemistries (*see* **Notes 7** and **8**.)

Vacuum Valve: A pneumatically actuated solenoid valve is used to isolate the chamber from the Vacuum Pump. The valve is opened to pump down to base pressure, purge, and closed to vent the Reaction Chamber to atmosphere.

Vent: As the process nears completion, the Reaction Chamber must be returned to atmospheric pressure in order to load and/or unload parts. This process is referred to as venting and begins with the closing of the Vacuum Valve. The Vent Routine begins with an optional slow vent function. The slow vent allows a neutral gas or air to leak into the system for a programmed length of time. After that point the main Vent Valve opens and room air enters the Reaction Chamber at maximum speed until the system has returned to atmospheric pressure.

View Port: The view port is a glass portal, with UV and RF filters, that enables viewing and monitoring of the plasma color and parts inside the Reaction Chamber (*see* **Note 6**). There are also view ports on the pumping station for observing and monitoring fluid levels.

Base Pressure: Base pressure refers to a set point whose function is to act as a pressure switch for a programmed process step. Equipment safety interlocks should be designed to ensure that the gases and the energy cannot be activated manually or automatically unless the system has reached the Base Pressure. A base pressure is selected that is lower that the processing pressure to ensure adequate evaluation of the chamber of out gassed species and moisture. Depending on the material, extended "pump downs" may be desirable to extend the out gassing step (*see* **Note 4**.)

Step: A step is defined as a discreet duration of time when the plasma process gases flow with or without energy. A series of steps makes up the complete process. A process may be comprised of multiple steps, allowing an operator to execute a recipe with different steps with a single process. For example, a part may be cleaned in Step A with one chemistry and activated in Step B with another chemistry, without removing the samples or venting to atmosphere.

Torr: A unit of pressure approximately equivalent to the pressure required to raise mercury up a tube one millimeter. There are 760 Torr in one atmosphere.

The relationship between different vacuum units is given here:

1,000 Torr

=0.00131 ATM (atmospheres)

=0.9999 mm Hg (millimeters of mercury)

=0.535 in. of H_2O

=0.0193 psi

760 Torr = 1 ATM

3   Methods

Plasma is referred to as the fourth state of matter. It is comprised of electrons, ions, and other excited meta-stables (*see* Fig. 3). The color of the plasma is distinct for every gas (*see* **Note 6**). The signature wavelengths of light are produced when excited electrons return back into a lower energy state. The spectra of light emissions will extend past the visible region into the UV and far UV. UV emissions can contribute to the surface modifications. This requires that chamber view ports are equipped with a UV filter. Substrates placed within the glow region are referred to as being within the "Primary" plasma. "Secondary" plasma refers to dark space regions outside the glow. The terms "downstream" or "remote" also refer to secondary plasma. The secondary plasma contains lower concentrations of charged species. The authors primarily practice surface modification within the primary plasma where there is a greater reactivity.

During the plasma process, energetic particles commence to cleave or form complexes with chemical bonds near the substrate surface. Unstable bonds and free radicals are produced on the substrate. They eventually recombine with molecular fragments or other charged moieties moving through the plasma. The dominant reaction on most polymer substrates occurs through hydrogen substitution along a polymer's aliphatic linkages. In the presence of oxygen, many hydrogen bonds are abstracted from the carbon backbone and then substituted by oxygen to form polar compounds.

Different chemical functionalities are produced by regulating the concentration of elements present within the plasma. Under these conditions the substrate material will form new covalent bonds and thereby the surface chemistry becomes reengineered. The chemical reactions generated by the plasma are generally confined to the substrate surface. The bulk properties are rarely impacted.

RF and microwaves sources efficiently generate plasma under partial vacuum pressure. Low gas pressures increase the mean free path allowing particles to accelerate with greater ease within the electromagnetic field. Collisions become less frequent translating to less heat generation from friction. Eventually particles do collide. There are both elastic and inelastic collisions. In an elastic collision the particle rebounds without losing or giving up its energy. It then continues to travel until its next collision. In an inelastic collision the particle gives up its energy and returns to its ground state (*see* Fig. 3). Within the primary plasma there is a continuous field for particles to accelerate within. This enables treatment of porous and microporous media such as filters, membranes, sintered parts, non-wovens, and foams. Reactive plasma species sustain enough energy to modify interstitial surfaces. [2]

3.1 Plasma Process Design

There exists a misconception that plasma processing provides a standard or universal result. The outcome of the plasma process will actually vary as a function of substrate material, chemistry selection, and many other factors related to the plasma process and equipment design. The following section identifies a methodology for designing, testing, and scaling a plasma process which produces a set of objectives.

1. *Problem definition*: Identify the project goals with a detailed account of the desired surface properties. Surface chemistry alone may not address all the material challenges. Consider other factors which may influence your result: surface topography, environment, processing aids, packaging, and sterilization. It may be possible to simultaneously address multiple surface property needs using a plasma process (*see* **Notes 1** and **2**)

2. *Equipment selection*: There are many options and system configurations which should be reviewed early in a project development. Note that a plasma process does not inherently scale or transfer from one equipment format to another. As an example, the research done in a small benchtop tool may not necessarily achieve an identical response in a reel-to-reel or larger batch system. The electrode size, spacing, orientation, and power source selection, influence the density and composition produced by the plasma. When possible utilize an equipment configuration that most closely matches the final size or desired equipment format. Realistically many opt for development or proof of concept in a small scale plasma system.

In this scenario keep a detailed record of the equipment used and coordinate project milestones with equipment transfer.

3. *Surface preparation*: Plasma interactions described herein predominantly occur on the sub-micron or atomic scales. Physical debris and contaminants that migrate to the surface may compromise the outcome of a surface modification. Remove undesirable species from the surface using appropriate cleaning methods. Only use solvents or detergents that are compatible with the material system. Additionally the surface should be properly rinsed of residual cleaning agents (*see* **Note 1**.)

4. *Plasma cleaning*: A short plasma cleaning step will help to ensure that a substrate surface becomes atomically clean. Organic oligomers and low molecular weight molecules are quickly deconstructed and removed by oxygen plasma. The recommended times for a plasma cleaning step vary, from a few seconds to a few minutes. Different gases, or combination of gases, may be selected to create desired plasma energies for ablating species. Table 2 lists examples of gases and vapors that

Table 2
Available gases and liquids for plasma chemistry applications

Gas	Liquids (create vapors)
Oxygen	Methanol
Argon	Water
Helium	Allylamine
Nitrogen	Ethylenediamine
Hydrogen	Acrylic acid
Nitrous oxide	Acetone
Carbon dioxide	Hydroxyethylmethacrylate
Air	Fluoroacrylates
Methane	Ethanol
Ethane	Toluene
Ethylene	Diaminopropane
Acetylene	Butylamine
Tetrafluoromethane	Glutaraldehyde
Hexafluoroethane	Hexamethyldisiloxane, Octamethylcyclotetrasiloxane Tetramethylsilane
Hexafluoropropylene	Polyethylene glycols
	Diglymes
	Silanes (amino, carboxy, hydroxyl, mercapto, vinyl)

may be used in a partial vacuum plasma reactor and used routinely by Plasmatreat for process development. For example, a mixture of oxygen and tetrafluoromethane produces more aggressive plasma. With judicious selection of conditions, expect no observable change to the substrate resulting from the plasma cleaning. Over treatment of polymeric materials could result in damage to the part. Surface ashing or hazing may be mitigated by reducing the power and/or treatment time. Furthermore a poor adhesion or a poor treatment stability could also be an indication of over treatment.

5. *Surface chemistry:* Plasma surface activation provides permanent and covalent attachment of surface chemistry. Chemical species are selectable by the gas and the vapor chemistry introduced into the plasma (*see* Table 2), resulting in unique functional species as shown in Fig. 4 and further described below.

(a) *Hydroxyl chemistry:* Gas plasma containing oxygen gas or alcohol vapor such methanol produce a sufficient density of surface hydroxyl groups. Hydroxyl groups link biological molecules through simple dehydration reactions. These also impart surface polarity which enhances substrate wettability. The simplicity of hydroxylation makes it one of the most common plasma modifications.

(b) *Carboxyl chemistry:* Gas plasma containing, carbon dioxide gas, acetic acid vapor, or acrylic acid vapor is used to produce carboxyl groups. The carboxylic acid functionality is an integral part of amino acids and it is especially useful in biomolecule capture. Under high pH the carboxylic acid will disassociate to form a carboxylate ion. Carboxyl surfaces are hydrophilic, are negatively charged, and are capable of nonspecific binding.

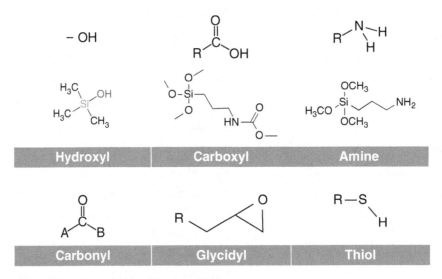

Fig. 4 Examples of plasma created functional species

(c) *Amine chemistry:* Gas plasma containing ammonia gas, diamine vapor, or allylamine vapor produce primary, secondary, and tertiary amine. Primary amines donate hydrogen atoms to form hydrogen bonds. Amines are commonly employed in the capture, immobilization, and retention of biological molecules such as proteins, lipids, and antibodies.

(d) *Custom chemistry:* Plasma processing enables many other possibilities in surface chemistry. Judicious selection of the gas and vapor species enables an operator to design and customize their surface chemistry to include deposition of thin film coatings, by the process known as Plasma Enhanced Chemical Vapor Deposition (PECVD). Example PECVD surfaces include hydrophobic and low retention coatings that may be used for dispensing components (*see* Table 1). The plasma contains many reactive and charged moieties that can change and alter the chemistries being input as gas or vapor. Ultimately the surface will form a distribution of chemical groups.

3.2 Process Development

The primary variables to study in a plasma process development program are: chemistry, gas and/or liquid vapor flow (resulting in specific pressures), plasma power, and process time. Keep in mind that polymers are complex and may express different affinities or susceptibilities to various plasma gases or plasma compositions (*see* **Note 1**). Therefore an implementation that worked with one material system will not inherently work with all material systems. A basic methodology for determining a successful plasma condition would be to screen plasma chemistry and then to optimize around a desirable surface response. A review of considerations in designing a process follows.

1. *Chemistry screening:* Process development begins with a screening of different plasma gas and vapor chemistries (*see* Table 2) with the objective of determining which plasma chemistries provide the greatest improvement in surface properties. Process chemistries which exhibit the most notable improvements become process candidates for further development and optimization. For example, a development in designing surface amine might compare the effectiveness of the following different plasma compositions: ammonia, argon with allylamine, and argon with aminopropyltrimethoxysilane. All of these processes are expected to deliver amine to the surface however the chemistry screening will determine which plasma chemistries best modify the substrate for the particular application. The ammonia process might yield a sufficient density of amine but that amine might be difficult to access because it resides as a pendant side group close to the polymer back bone.

The allylamine on the other hand may form short chains or even a branched structure influencing steric hindrance (*see* Fig. 4.) The plasma chemistry screening practically tests the substrates susceptibility to plasma and provides insights into unique surface properties traits that might otherwise remain undefined.

2. *Process optimization:* The density of surface chemistry, the coating thickness, network structure and hydrophobic effect are some of the properties that may be fine-tuned during process optimization. Process improvements are made by investigating variations in the plasma parameters. For example, once the chemistry has been identified in the screening phase, a Box-Behnken design of experiment provides an effective architecture for experimental design. The primary variables affecting the process design at this stage are power, time and gas ratio. The plasma power and process time will usually impact the density of surface chemistry and stability of the treatment. If the plasma power becomes too intense then the gas species fragment and lead to performance loss. At low power the density or concentration of surface functionality might be too low and this would also manifest in decreased performance. In addition to the primary variables noted, pulsed power plasma and/or modified duty cycles may be employed for control of branching, fragmentation, surface roughness and temperature management. In one example of process development, an argon and acrylic acid plasma produced a functional density of carboxyl groups on a porous membrane. Although suitable surface conjugation was demonstrated during the screening study the treatment increased hydrophobicity of the membrane resulting in poor membrane flux. To optimize the process oxygen was added into the plasma. This improved the wettability of the surface treatment. An oxygen flow was determined that improved membrane flux. This did not negatively impact the effectiveness of the carboxyl species.

3. *Gas or vapor flow:* The concentration and composition of the plasma chemistry affects the generation of surface chemistry. Flow management systems (such as MFCs and LFCs described in Subheading 2) will regulate and ideally monitor flow into the plasma chamber. Vapor chemistries are typically accompanied by a co-process gas. They will assist in sustaining a uniform glow. Inert gases such as argon and helium make good candidates for co-process gas because they do not form chemical bonds with the primary gas chemistry. Oxygen containing compounds will have a tendency to oxidize other species within the chamber. This may be undesirable in an example where the projected amine would be converted to an undesired nitrogen oxide. The gas flow into chamber volumes less than 5 cubic feet generally does not exceed one liter per minute. Liquid flows in vapor delivery systems do not generally exceed 20 ml/h.

4. *Chamber pressure*: The process pressure affects the process temperature and the plasma density. The process pressure usually results from the flow of species into the reactor chamber. Regulating pressure independent of flow is not necessary, however some process chemists favor controlling the chamber pressure by adjusting pump impedance at the vacuum port using a throttle valve (*see* **Note 5**.) Higher pressure plasma processes generally contain more thermal energy whereas lower pressure plasma contains more energetic species.

5. *Continuous vs. pulsed power*: Plasma power is one of the most notable influences on the surface modification. Some plasma generators come with the ability to pulse the power and to employ a duty cycle. Pulse and duty cycle enable an operator to reduce plasma temperature. This is especially critical in the modification of thermally sensitive materials. Plasma temperatures may also introduce surface stress which could negatively impacts treatment stability in some material systems. Pulse and duty cycle are valuable tools in plasma film formation such as the deposition of ultra-thin coatings. This works by regulating kinetic events within the polymerization reaction. The power cycles have the ability to influence coating thickness, coating chemistry, and coating density.

6. *Interstitial modification*: Partial vacuum plasma processing is advantageous for modifying the interstices of porous media, in addition to the visible outer surfaces. This technique is ideal for changing the wicking and binding properties of sintered, woven, non-woven, and membrane materials that are commonly used for filtration (*see* Table 1). As described herein, the equipment used creates primary plasma. In primary plasma, there is a greater mean free path of the particles before a collision. This sustained energy is ideal for modifying the interstices of porous media, or for use inside complex nano-scale vias or channels. With atmospheric processes, on the other hand, the mean free path is short when the species are out of the direct energy field, thus the treatment area is limited. The first step of the process, where modification in either the inner dimensions or interstices is required, requires conditions to ensure that the polymer is out gassed. In all plasma processes, the reaction occurs between the plasma and surface. Removing barriers from the surface is critical for a successful modification. In a vacuum process, the first step is the pump down phase, which is further described in Subheading 3.3. During an out gassing step, extended time for the pump down as well as a lower based pressure is important (*see* **Note 4**). Following the pump down, the plasma may be introduced continuously or via multiple step process. An example of the wicking and wetting effect of a high density polyethylene, following an oxygen plasma

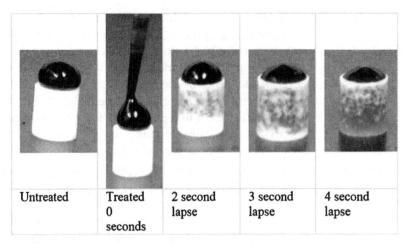

| Untreated | Treated 0 seconds | 2 second lapse | 3 second lapse | 4 second lapse |

Fig. 5 Interstitial modification of porous media for enhanced wicking

process, is shown in Fig. 5. With judicious selection of plasma processing parameters, surface stability may result in years of storage prior to use.

3.3 Plasma Treatment in Partial Vacuum System

Once a study has been outlined, the steps to partial vacuum processing are simply listed as follows:

1. The components, to be treated, are placed in the Reactor Chamber, which is vacated, via a pumping system, to a base pressure that may range from 25 to 100 mtorr (*see* **Note 4**). During this initial processing step, the isolation valve is in the open position.

2. Process gas(es) and/or liquid vapors are introduced into the chamber at a desired flow rate to attain a specific pressure (*see* **Note 3**).

3. RF energy (as used in the Plasma Science, PTS and Plasmatreat partial vacuum systems) is supplied to electrodes within the chamber and excites the vapors/gas (es) into a plasma (*see* **Note 3**).

4. During processing, pressure is continuously monitored as an indicator of chemistry uniformity (*see* **Notes 6–8**).

5. While under vacuum a sequence of multiple steps may be conducted as part of a single recipe. Between each step and after the last step the chamber is pumped down to the base pressure to evacuate gases from the previous step (*see* **Notes 4** and **8**).

6. Following completion of the last step, there is a venting cycle in either room air or a neutral gas such as nitrogen, to bring the chamber to atmosphere. The venting speed is controlled to minimize disruption to fragile components, if required.

7. The parts are removed and packaged or transferred to a subsequent process (*see* **Note 2**).

**3.4 Evaluation
of Plasma Treated
Surface**

Designing a validation method is as important as designing the plasma process. It is critical to validate the surface with a test that is representative and correlates to your application. A few popular techniques for quantifying and qualifying the effects of a plasma surface modification are described herein.

1. *Surface energy*: The alteration to the surface bonds will usually change the surface tension. Contact angle and dyne inks provide a means for rapid examination for surface tensions. Water will generally form lower contact angles on polar surfaces. The contact angles are measured between the substrate and the tangent where the droplet meets the surface. Only use distilled water when making a water contact angle measurement. Low surface wetting angles correlate well with oxygen functionalities. Surface dyne inks come in kits containing numerous fluids with differing surface tension. A dyne fluid must have a lower surface energy in order to wet onto a surface. Otherwise the fluid will bead up or retract. The surface dyne method and the water contact angle provide a facile methodology for probing the plasma treated surface. Note that these methods do not necessarily discriminate chemical functionality. Surface energy probes such as dyne level and water contact angle do not make successful engineering specification. The authors recommend using such surface analysis methods as process quality control tools if results may be validated by functional testing.

2. *Chemical analysis*: There are numerous analytical tools which are able to determine a surface's chemical composition. Some examples include X-ray Photoelectron Spectroscopy (XPS), Nuclear Magnetic Resonance (NMR), Time-of-Flight Secondary Ion Mass Spectrometry (TOF SIMS) and Energy Dispersive Spectroscopy (EDS). These and similar methods are useful in attributing surface affects to the fundamental surface chemistry. Unfortunately many of these methods are not readily available due to cost and requirement of trained specialists, and their results do not necessarily predict success. Analytical methods make useful research tools in plasma surface engineering.

3. *Markers/Stains*: Staining and fluorescent probe methods are especially useful in evaluating the surface. Testing is highly functional and typically relevant to the application. A successful conjugation will show good retention after washing. Evaluate the surface for good selectivity and a low coefficient of variation. Low retention could be an indication of a poor surface chemistry or a problem with surface contamination. A high coefficient of variation could indicate poor chamber uniformity or again a surface contaminant.

4. *Stability and Accelerated Aging*: Treatment stability should be assessed for every application. Many of the reactive surface

chemistries are sensitive to environmental effects. These effects could include moisture, temperature, light, exposure to solvents and oxidation. If the parts need to be stored use a clean packaging material. Most plastic bags contain plasticizer or anti-blocking agents that will confound a plasma surface treatment (*see* **Notes 1** and **2**). The authors use heat sealable forensics bags for short term storage. Polymer substrates are especially prone to surface changes over time. In general the surface treatment will diminish quickly on low durometer elastomers and on materials with low glass transition temperatures. Mobile surfaces lose surface treatment to reorientation more quickly than a glassy surface. Accelerated aging may be used to simulate long term stability. Most polymer systems adhere to the rule of time-temperature superposition allowing thermal analysts to extrapolate time dependent behavior using heat. Large deviations occur from real world behavior when extrapolating too far out or when performing accelerated aging with improper conditions.

4 Notes

When designing a plasma process, take into consideration the equipment operation, base material, design of the process and subsequent environment. Once a plasma chemistry has been targeted, if you observe irregular results (uneven treatment), consider further examination of the surface cleaning and preparation step as well as placement of the part(s) in the chamber. With some processes, rotating the part may be required to ensure even treatment.

1. Variables in material may impact the performance of plasma treated surfaces. Therefore it is important to define your material and material manufacturing before starting plasma surface treatment. A change in polymers and/or manufacturing techniques may impact the process. Variables include:

   (a) Additives (stabilizers, pigments, nucleating agents, plasticizers) and the propensity for migration of additives.

   (b) Propensity for molecular rotation.

   (c) Finishes.

   (d) Mold release materials.

   (e) Machining debris.

   (f) Moisture retain/absorption/adsorption.

   (g) Cleanliness (and how is the substrate cleaned prior to plasma).

   (h) Potential for oxidation.

2. Subsequent steps post process can impact the performance of the plasma treated surface. These may include:

    (a) Adhesive techniques (bonding, heat sealing, ultrasonic welding).

    (b) Chemical exposure.

    (c) Cleaning and/or sterilization processes.

    (d) Careful material handling to eliminate the transfer or contamination of plasma treated product.

    (e) Monitoring selection of glove type and compatibility of the glove materials with chemicals.

    (f) Storage selection and proper packaging material is important to limit plasma treated surface contamination.

    (g) Temperature and light exposure

3. Power and gas flow deficiencies should be monitored. If the equipment used is manually controlled or lacks capabilities to define set points for a given component, carefully monitor the output device. Monitoring with a secondary calibrated tool may be required. Be cognoscente of reflected power where the programmed power is not actually delivered to the electrodes.

4. When designing a process, choosing the base pressure is important. Too high of a base pressure may impact the out gassing process. Base pressure should always be below your operating pressure to ensure our gassing of the part and chamber. The chamber may absorb moisture during non-use. Careful monitoring of the time to reach base pressure in an empty chamber and a chamber with parts is an important step in designing the process and ensuring consistent results.

5. Once the process has been developed and fixturing optimized, take great care to observe and monitor the pressure. A change in the pressure is a signal that a component may not be working per specification and/or there is chamber or part contamination. Note that some plasma equipment includes a throttle valve. A throttle valve, "throttles" the pumping capacity of the chamber, which modifies the pressure of the species inside the chamber. Equipment supplied with automated throttle valves work by changing this throttle (thus vacuum conductance) to meet a pressure set point. This maintains a constant pressure in the chamber by adjusting the vacuum conductance. When using a throttle valve, be sure to check the health of your pumping system and flow controllers as the condition may be masked due to the automatic adjustment.

6. One of the simplest ways to monitor the plasma process is by observing the plasma color. A change in color may be indicative of gas flow issues, air leaks, excessive out gassing or an unclean chamber.

7. The nature of the vacuum plasma process introduces new species. These species may deposit on the inner surfaces of the chamber, thus design of a chamber cleaning protocol ensures reproducible results. This includes manually wiping the chamber of dust; cleaning the exposed surface between the chamber and isolation valve, and a plasma process to remove organic build up.

8. Regularly perform maintenance checks to ensure that there are not any slow leaks due to loose fittings or worn sealing surfaces. It is important to maintain a log of daily (or weekly) checks to monitor both the pump down speed and leak up rate of the chamber with and without parts. A drift in either of these conditions is an immediate warning of either a system issue or materials issue.

References

1. Plasma Science and Plasma Technology Systems Equipment Operations Manual Glossary Section, 1997 through 2015

2. Plasma Science, Technical Note 7, October 1989

INDEX

Robert Hnasko (ed.), *ELISA: Methods and Protocols*, Methods in Molecular Biology, vol. 1318,
DOI 10.1007/978-1-4939-2742-5, © Springer Science+Business Media New York 2015

CPSIA information can be obtained at www.ICGtesting.com
Printed in the USA
LVOW05*0911120715

445930LV00004B/64/P